Pastoral Care
of the Mentally Disabled:
Advancing Care
of the Whole Person

Pastoral Care
of the Mentally Disabled:
Advancing Care
of the Whole Person

Sally K. Severino, MD
The Reverend Richard Liew, PhD
Editors

The Haworth Pastoral Press
An Imprint of
The Haworth Press, Inc.
New York · London · Norwood (Australia)

r'

Published by

The Haworth Pastoral Press, 10 Alice Street, Binghamton, NY 13904-1580 USA

The Haworth Pastoral Press is an imprint of The Haworth Press, Inc., 10 Alice Street, Binghamton, NY 13904-1580 USA

Pastoral Care of the Mentally Disabled: Advancing Care of the Whole Person has also been published as *Journal of Religion in Disability & Rehabilitation*, Volume 1, Number 2 1994.

The development, preparation, and publication of this work has been undertaken with great care. However, the publisher, employees, editors, and agents of The Haworth Press and all imprints of The Haworth Press, Inc., including The Haworth Medical Press and Pharmaceutical Products Press, are not responsible for any errors contained herein or for consequences that may ensue from use of materials or information contained in this work. Opinions expressed by the author(s) are not necessarily those of The Haworth Press, Inc.

The Haworth Press, Inc., 10 Alice Street, Binghamton, NY 13904-1580 USA

Library of Congress Cataloging-in-Publication Data

Pastoral care of the mentally disabled: advancing care of the whole person / Sally K. Severino, Richard Liew, editors.
     p. cm.
Includes bibliographical references.
ISBN 1-56024-665-0 (alk. paper)
     1. Church work with the mentally ill. 2. Mentally ill–Pastoral counseling of. 3. Mental illness–Treatment. 4. Psychiatry. I. Severino, Sally K. II. Liew, Richard.
BV4461.P27 1994
259'.4-dc20
94–17287
CIP

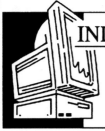

INDEXING & ABSTRACTING

Contributions to this publication are selectively indexed or abstracted in print, electronic, online, or CD-ROM version(s) of the reference tools and information services listed below. This list is current as of the copyright date of this publication. See the end of this section for additional notes.

- *Abstracts in Anthropology,* Baywood Publishing Company, 26 Austin Avenue, P. O. Box 337, Amityville, NY 11701

- *Abstracts of Research in Pastoral Care & Counseling,* Loyola College, 7135 Minstrel Way, Suite 101, Columbia, MD 21045

- *Applied Social Sciences Index & Abstracts (ASSIA),* Bowker-Saur Limited, Maypole House, Maypole Road, East Grinstead, West Sussex RH19 1HH, England

- *Cumulative Index to Nursing & Allied Health Literature (CINAHL),* CINAHL Information Systems, P. O. Box 871/1509 Wilson Terrace, Glendale, CA 91209

- *Human Resources Abstracts,* Sage Publications, Inc., 2455 Teller Road, Newbury Park, CA 91320

- *Occupational Therapy Index,* British Library Medical Information Service, Boston Spa, Wetherby, West Yorkshire LS23 7BQ, United Kingdom

- *Periodica Islamica,* Berita Publishing, 22 Jalan Liku, 59100 Kuala Lumpur, Malaysia

- *Sage Family Studies Abstracts,* Sage Publications, Inc., 2455 Teller Road, Newbury Park, CA 91320

- *Theology Digest (also made available on CD-ROM),* St. Louis University, 3650 Lindell Boulevard, St. Louis, MO 63108

(continued)

SPECIAL BIBLIOGRAPHIC NOTES

related to special journal issues (separates)
and indexing/abstracting

☐ indexing/abstracting services in this list will also cover material in the "separate" that is co-published simultaneously with Haworth's special thematic journal issue or DocuSerial. Indexing/abstracting usually covers material at the article/chapter level.

☐ monographic co-editions are intended for either non-subscribers or libraries which intend to purchase a second copy for their circulating collections.

☐ monographic co-editions are reported to all jobbers/wholesalers/approval plans. The source journal is listed as the "series" to assist the prevention of duplicate purchasing in the same manner utilized for books-in-series.

☐ to facilitate user/access services all indexing/abstracting services are encouraged to utilize the co-indexing entry note indicated at the bottom of the first page of each article/chapter/contribution.

☐ this is intended to assist a library user of any reference tool (whether print, electronic, online, or CD-ROM) to locate the monographic version if the library has purchased this version but not a subscription to the source journal.

☐ individual articles/chapters in any Haworth publication are also available through the Haworth Document Delivery Services (HDDS).

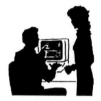

Pastoral Care of the Mentally Disabled: Advancing Care of the Whole Person

CONTENTS

Symposium Proceedings, The New York Hospital-Cornell Medical Center/Westchester Division with The Hospital Chaplaincy, Inc. and The American Association of Pastoral Counselors (Eastern Region)

ALL HAWORTH PASTORAL PRESS
BOOKS AND JOURNALS ARE PRINTED
ON CERTIFIED ACID-FREE PAPER

ABOUT THE EDITORS

Sally K. Severino, MD, is Associate Professor of Clinical Psychiatry at Cornell University Medical College, and Associate Medical Director for Program Development and Director of Evaluation and Admissions Service for the New York Hospital, Westchester Division. She has a long-standing interest in psychiatry and religion and has been a member of the Committee on Psychiatry and Religion of the Group for the Advancement of Psychiatry since 1984.

The Reverend Richard Liew, PhD, is Director of Pastoral Care & Education at New York Hospital-Cornell University Medical Center/ Westchester Division, in White Plains, New York. He has held a private practice in individual and group psychotherapy and marital and family counseling since 1974. Dr. Liew is a member of many professional societies and is a Diplomate in the American Association of Pastoral Couselors and a Fellow in the College of Chaplains.

Preface

There is growing public interest in bringing religion from the periphery to the center of society. Both psychiatrists and clergy can assist people in this process, but the process demands a continuing dialogue between the two disciplines. It is hoped that this material will facilitate a dialogue between clergy and mental health professionals that will encourage a partnership towards evaluating and treating patients with mental illness.

To accomplish this goal, sixteen participants joined together on May 13, 1992 in a day-long symposium to begin the dialogue. The symposium was sponsored by The New York Hospital-Cornell Medical Center/Westchester Division with The Hospital Chaplaincy, Inc. and The American Association of Pastoral Counselors (Eastern Region).

The role of the church is perceived to be about spirituality. The role of the mental hospital is perceived to be about caring for the mentally ill. This decade calls for the participation of both the church and the hospital in the process of healing the mentally ill. For this to occur, the certainties of the perceived roles of clergy and physician must be questioned. New information must be shared and accepted by those in each discipline. New tasks must be developed. Only in this way can psychiatrists and clergy move beyond narrowly defined roles to partnership roles in the process of healing.

We thank the Josiah Macy, Jr. Foundation and the Upjohn Company for their help and support in enabling this work to develop.

Sally K. Severino, MD
The Reverend Richard Liew, PhD

[Haworth co-indexing entry note]: "Preface." Severino, Sally K., and The Reverend Richard Liew. Co-published simultaneously in the *Journal of Religion in Disability & Rehabilitation* (The Haworth Press, Inc.) Vol. 1, No. 2, 1994, p. xiii; and: *Pastoral Care of the Mentally Disabled: Advancing Care of the Whole Person* (ed: Sally K. Severino, and The Reverend Richard Liew) The Haworth Press, Inc., 1994, p. xi. Multiple copies of this article/chapter may be purchased from The Haworth Document Delivery Center [1-800-3-HAWORTH; 9:00 a.m. - 5:00 p.m. (EST)].

xi

Introduction

Sally K. Severino, MD

Mending the mind (medicine) and minding the soul (ministry) are both essential for healing. Healing can best occur when these two, mind and soul/medicine and ministry, are yoked. That is what this volume intends to address.

Currently, the pathophysiology of disease is better understood than the process of healing. The process of healing, that is, the internal mechanisms of mind, body and soul (such as the immune system) that repairs disease, continues to mystify us. Yet clinically we continually observe that love, hope and faith contribute to healing. Conversely, loss of love, hope and faith can and often does contribute to illness.

Observation of this process is not new. The sixteenth-century physician, Paracelsus, wrote of the invisible aspects of healing. He declared, "Man has a visible and an invisible workshop. The visible one is his body, the invisible one is imagination (mind). . . . The imagination is the sun in the soul of man. . . . The spirit is the master, imagination the tool, and the body the plastic material. . . . The power of the imagination is a great factor in medicine. It may produce diseases in man and animals and it may cure it. . . . Ills of the body may be cured by physical remedies or by the power of the spirit acting through the soul" (Hartmann, 1973, p. 112).

More recently (1876-1965) Anton Boisen exemplified in his life the synthesis of medicine and ministry in healing. He was the first mental hospital chaplain in the United States and a founder of the movement providing clinical training for clergy in health care settings. He, him-

[Haworth co-indexing entry note]: "Introduction." Severino, Sally K. Co-published simultaneously in the *Journal of Religion in Disability & Rehabilitation* (The Haworth Press, Inc.) Vol. 1, No. 2, 1994, pp. 1-2; and: *Pastoral Care of the Mentally Disabled: Advancing Care of the Whole Person* (ed: Sally K. Severino, and The Reverend Richard Liew) The Haworth Press, Inc., 1994, pp. 1-2. Multiple copies of this article/chapter may be purchased from The Haworth Document Delivery Center [1-800-3-HA-WORTH; 9:00 a.m. - 5:00 p.m. (EST)].

self, suffered from mental illness. Boisen felt he derived religious insight into mental disorder from his experience which he then shared with ministers and theological students whom he taught and supervised. Boisen's example may be likened to the "creative illness" of others whose major achievements followed similar patterns of struggle.

REFERENCE

Hartmann, Franz. *The Life and Teachings of Paracelsus*. Blauvelt, New York: Rudolf Steiner Publications, 1973.

The Role of Faith in Mental Healing: Psychoanalysis and Faith

Harold Bronheim, MD

Despite the diversity of psychoanalytic perspectives pursued worldwide, the most significant clinical debate over many years has occurred between proponents of classical drive-oriented, conflict/defense theory and proponents of modern self-psychological deficit-based theory (Tuttman, 1987; Aron, 1990). This debate is a reflection of a larger philosophical approach argued between advocates of part mechanisms developing into whole psychic entities and advocates of synthetic wholes breaking into symptomatic parts. Although it is commonly believed that theory and technique develop concurrently, in fact, psychoanalytic technique pursues an inexorable development that usually receives theoretical justification only after the fact (Jackel, 1966). Technically, many practitioners utilize a flexible approach, simultaneously incorporating both poles of the theoretical spectrum in their analytic investigation.

Nevertheless, many analysts have had the regular experience of their most carefully crafted interpretations, exquisitely timed, falling on deaf ears, and other spontaneous comments or interactions producing profound reactions and precipitating breakthroughs to new states of awareness. It is as if growth and, by extension, cure come about to a significant degree in an unpredictable, discontinuous fashion through some interactions with an unknown factor in the mind of the patient or in the relationship with the analyst.

[Haworth co-indexing entry note]: "The Role of Faith in Mental Healing: Psychoanalysis and Faith." Bronheim, Harold. Co-published simultaneously in the *Journal of Religion in Disability & Rehabilitation* (The Haworth Press, Inc.) Vol. 1, No. 2, 1994, pp. 3-18; and: *Pastoral Care of the Mentally Disabled: Advancing Care of the Whole Person* (ed: Sally K. Severino, and The Reverend Richard Liew) The Haworth Press, Inc., 1994, pp. 3-18. Multiple copies of this article/chapter may be purchased from The Haworth Document Delivery Center [1-800-3-HAWORTH; 9:00 a.m. - 5:00 p.m. (EST)].

3

Faith also is a frequently encountered and inexplicable experience in mental life. It can appear suddenly in the communications of our patients and, unfortunately, all too often is passed over by us. Patients who profess to have strong religious beliefs often have little real faith, and others with little religious feeling are strongly faithful. By and large, psychoanalysis has dealt with faith in theory only and has avoided it in clinical practice. Therefore, we will endeavor to understand faith and its relationship to psychoanalytic theory, its contribution through its absence to aggression, and its necessity for growth in analysis.

Considering its importance, it is noteworthy how psychoanalysis has distanced itself from the study of faith, and has dealt with it, for the most part, in theory only. According to Freud, religious ideas are "not the precipitates of experience or end results of our thinking, but illusions, fulfillments of the oldest, strongest and most urgent wishes of mankind. The secret of their strength lies in the strength of those wishes" (Freud, 1961, p. 30). Although this is most certainly true with regard to most aspects of religion, it does not necessarily apply to the more important areas of faith.

Following upon Freud, in the American ego-psychology school, religious faith has been viewed as the outcome of the Oedipal situation. It is a superego development whose aim is to deal with sexual and aggressive wishes. In it we recognize reaction formation, love and submission to a beneficent God instead of hatred of the feared father, as well as compulsive rituals. In addition, we recognize the central role of biblical myths such as the near-sacrifice of Isaac or the actual crucifixion of Christ, both of which involve fantasies of father/child murders (Mann, 1962).

Following upon Klein in the British object relations school, Winnicott saw the evolving experience of self not so much as a defense against anxiety and the resolution of conflict, but as an original sense of joy and rapture in the movement from transitional object to object usage (Eigen, 1981). Faith and its associated affects flow directly from this early developmental leap. Balint (1968) was also concerned about a "basic fault" that appeared in the psychopathology of his patients that needed to be traversed in a leap in the analytic process.

For Bion, faith is an even earlier mystical experience that begins in development as an absolute belief in the object called "O." It can be experienced but never known. He draws upon a distinction between being and knowing that although inextricably linked are qualitatively different (Eigen, 1985). For Bion the emotional truth in analysis turns on this point and cure evolves out of this personal experience.

Despite the recognition over the years that faith is an essential emotional state, there has been little formal application of it in psychoanalytic technique or systematic investigation of its significance in bringing about cure.

RELIGIOUS FAITH AND OBJECT RELATIONS

Martin Buber, a pre-eminent Jewish philosopher of the twentieth century, relates the following tale of the Hasidic Rabbi Shneur Zalman, of Northern White Russia, Belarus (died in 1813). Rabbi Zalman was denounced to the authorities and ultimately executed. While in jail he was approached by the chief of the gendarmes, who asked, "How are we to understand that God, the all-knowing, said to Adam 'Where art thou?'" Rabbi Zalman answered the officer simply and directly that God's question, "Where art thou?", seeks to implore Adam to give an account of himself as to what he has been doing with his life, and how he has been hiding himself from the truth about himself. Rabbi Zalman went on to say that the question, although asked of Adam, is an eternal one for all men through every generation to examine the hideouts and falsehoods in each man's life and how he hides himself from the face of God. Adam's reply, "I was afraid and I hid myself," is not so much a submission or surrender to authority as it is an examination of the truths about himself that allowed a returning to God (Buber, 1966). Buber goes on to say that the question by God is a purposeful effort to get Adam and, therefore, man, to draw closer to God through the exploration of himself and his self-deceptions which pull him from his own true self.

How extraordinary a proposition it is of Buber and the Hasidic rabbis that man's ills, no matter how complex, independent of psychology, social situations, and biological temperament, flow directly from his disconnection with God! And furthermore, by giving account of oneself and by being able to say in effect, "Here I am," one is able once again to become at peace with himself and the world. It is in this leap of faith and movement back to God and therefore from a false to a true self that leads to cure. We recognize in it a rather interesting overlap with object relations theory as applied in clinical practice.

According to Kernberg, "Unconscious intrapsychic conflicts are never simply conflicts between impulses and defenses; rather the drive derivative finds expression through a certain primitive object relation (a certain unit of self-and-object representation); and the defense too is reflected by a certain internalized object relation. The conflict is between these intrapsychic structures" (Kernberg, 1980, p. 155).

Psychoanalysis (in the post-ego psychology era) involves an exploration of unconscious internal objects as they are projected onto the analyst within the transference, and an exploration of the ways in which patients resist those efforts to alter their perceptions despite the actual experience with the analyst (Ogden, 1984). Wallerstein (1988), in his survey of international variations in psychoanalytic technique, believes this to be the essential core of psychoanalysis. Our interpretations attempt to demonstrate to the patient the distortions created by the reexperience of his internal object relations. The resistance to change requires that the patient maintain a safe interpersonal distance while using other more primitive and inflexible mechanisms to cling to the object of the analyst. The analyst, through careful observation as well as empathic participation in the structured environment of the analytic dyad, encourages the patient to recognize and give up his resistance.

According to Gill (1982, pp. 26-27), "how much initiative the analyst will take in making transference interpretations depends on how ubiquitous he believes transference implications are in the patient's associations, how important he believes it is for these implications to become explicit, and how confident he is that they will spontaneously become explicit if he waits for this."

No matter what theoretical framework one begins with or which particular aspects one prefers to emphasize, successful technique leads to an active drawing of the analysand closer in self-object terms which can be observed and felt directly (by both parties) with the successive expression of intense affects originally attached to the more primitive internal self-objects. Are we not, therefore, in asking our analysands for their associations, saying to them, "Where art thou?" Are we not encouraging patients to reveal themselves and their hideouts, to give a true account of themselves? And is the patient not turning to us and allowing the emergence of the most intimate fears and feelings of shame when they admit, "I was afraid and I was hiding?"

Returning to the scriptures, we discover that this question by God to Adam is the first question asked in the Bible and occurs in Genesis immediately after the eating of the fruit of the "Tree of Knowledge." An alternative interpretation of this passage by rabbinic scholars of the past places God's question within the context of Genesis itself and speaks to another existential position. Just like life itself, consciousness and man's awareness of self involves God's immediate involvement and it is God's activity through his question and its penetration into his creation that brings forth consciousness.

Consciousness, being an attribute existing only in man, raises the question of its special origin; and it is argued that it is God's intervention through his question that precipitates its awareness. Eating fruit from the "Tree of Knowledge" is not in itself sufficient.

The passage in the Bible as it has been interpreted by rabbinic scholars, therefore, speaks to existential selves: one that is experiential and relational and the other that is more observational and rational. In it, we recognize the similarity to the duality of psychoanalytic technique moving at times between the poles of neutral-interpretive-observer and empathic-introspective participants (Tuttman, 1987).

According to Buber (1951) there are only two varieties of faith although there are many varieties in the contents of faith. One can have either faith in someone else without knowing why one should have it or else faith that something is true without knowing in fact that is so. For the theist, both varieties of faith coexist in the belief in a concept called God. Without factual evidence of it being so, the theist both believes in God's continuous existence and trusts in His beneficence. Although a believer may later maintain rational-appearing "proofs" of his position, they never occur *a priori*. God begins first in faith and is true regardless of proof. In fact, if there were proof, it would no longer be faith.

Developmental theory postulates that the self as distinct from object arises as a direct outcome of multiple mother/child interactions. At approximately 15-18 months of age, in Mahler's so-called rapprochment phase, the child becomes aware that mother is not only a source of security but actually a separate entity (Mahler, 1975). His attention shifts from locomotion and exploration to social interaction. Peek-a-boo games where the mother stimulates the child by hiding and calling out "Where are you?" to the delight of the child are played over and over again. Basic trust is the underlying relationship and the individuating child responds in time to the delightful and mysterious game of peek-a-boo by hiding itself in turn and then announcing in some fashion, "Here I am." It is remarkable that this game which reflects a milestone of self-object development is so reminiscent of the biblical question, "Where art thou?" and the response, "I was hiding."

Faith, it would seem, begins in the earliest phases of individuation, long before there is any certain awareness of self and obviously no awareness of religion. Reason and fact are relatively unimportant to the truth of faith and appear only as secondary elaborations to satisfy the needs of rationality. The power of faith stems from its origins in the early self-object relationship and many of its manifestations (idealization, omnipotence, splitting) as well as its penetration through the personality, reflect this early beginning. Faith, however, is not the same as basic trust. Faith is a trust that endures over time and physical separation. It is not sufficient for the developing child to recognize its self and object. It must also develop a sense of self and object constancy. Faith is the essential emotional state that enables a positive inner image of the object to be sustained irrespective of either satisfaction or dissatisfaction, and may undergo remodeling throughout the life cycle.

If there is an "illusion" to maintain, it is the illusion of object constancy. We currently think of object constancy as a stable quantity that remains solid once it is achieved. But object constancy, like faith, is a relative and fluid intrapsychic state and often requires remodeling and the use of transitional objects especially after periods of loss. Insofar as life is filled with loss, the intense grief that we experience in mourning may be in part the pain we suffer in giving up our illusion of secure and constant objects. Analysis itself is commonly interrupted by loss with no other work being able to be done at the time of loss except the work of mourning (Tarachow, 1963).

However, in the vast psychiatric literature on loss and grief there is little discussion about the appearance of faith. Yet so many of our patients have powerful resurgent feelings of faith at times of profound loss, including participation in religious rituals. Religious faith serves as a means to restore the lost object (even everlastingly) as it softens the reality and allows the gradual mastery of loss. Melancholia, on the other hand, may be the despair and disorganization experienced with the collapse of faith and the inner sense of bitter and irredeemable abandonment.

PSYCHOANALYTIC TECHNIQUE AND FAITH

It is unlikely that psychoanalytic cure occurs through intellectual awareness alone or a passive restructuring of the internal object relationships. Psychoanalysis is a dynamically engaged relationship that is mutually shared and bilaterally observed. It is an active process that directly involves us and even has profound effects on us, and when performed well, it leads to what Langs (1981) referred to as truth therapy. It is this active seeking of meaning by the patient with the participation of the analyst that prepares the patient for change. When hidden truths are uncovered in analysis, they are initially associated with affects that can be quite intense, and which only later are followed by a sense of well-being and security. These personal truths experienced within the trusting analytic dyad can be relied upon to provide a foundation for a leap of faith to self object constancy that cannot be found elsewhere in the patient's life.

Where religious faith appears in psychoanalysis, and it frequently does, a more vigorous examination of the affect (what it feels like and not necessarily the nature of its content or its rituals) can lead to valuable understanding of the unconscious conflicts and the deficits within the internal object relations.

Brief examples of the above from the therapy of religious individuals include one Hasidic woman with inflammatory bowel disease who stated quite early that she felt that God hated her. Over time, she was observed to have numerous histrionic traits and regularly abused drugs. After several years of testing and acting out, a history of sexual molestation at an early age was uncovered. Another elderly Catholic woman with heart disease who had a borderline personality with intense anger stated that God had abandoned her. She had lost her son at a young age and had never resolved the loss. She felt betrayed by God and prayed instead directly to her son whom she substituted for God. Another neurotically anxious Catholic woman who converted and married a Moslem man felt that God was one and the same and loved her however she referred to or named him, but she was very attached to her father, and unable to give him up while remaining only minimally attached to her husband. In each of these examples, a deeper examination of the nature of the patient's religious faith provided early important clues about the state of their conflicts and relationships to important objects.

In analysis, when we observe sudden and dramatic flights into health, we know them to be defensive positions behind which lie frightening if not overwhelming affects. They frequently account for impasses in the form of negative therapeutic reactions (Danielian and Lister, 1988). So, too, sudden religious conversions at times of great loss are to be viewed with great caution. Individuals so affected are under enormous tension and the defenses are unstable and often deteriorate over time.

Unfortunately, many patients, especially those with narcissistic, histrionic, and borderline features, express an amorphous feeling of void within themselves. In that void they feel totally alone and disconnected. As much as they might wish to, they feel distant from and unable to trust others, including the analyst. They also feel insecure on their own and unable to trust themselves. They not uncommonly report that they feel that the analyst disappears when they leave the session or at other times of affective lability. By actively engaging and empathically trying to understand the patient's painful inner experience, the void is transiently filled with the object of the analyst. The repetitive experience of trusting another human being while simultaneously working through and testing them with projective identification enables the patient to solidify a faith in the continuous existence of the relationship with the analyst and ultimately, therefore, in a synthetic sense of self.

A breach of faith on the other hand, even unintentionally on the part of the analyst, leads to injury and an increased sense of isolation for the patient. It inevitably leads to an "acting out" or a resistance to further work in therapy. The aggression that emerges is intended either as a direct retaliation for the injury that has been sustained or is a means to signal the analyst to proceed carefully in order to prevent any further disruption and disconnection from the object. The absence of faith or the threat of its loss, therefore, is a significant source of aggression in analysis.

PSYCHOANALYTIC FAITH OCCURS IN LEAPS

Although analysts generally agree upon what mix of psychological, interpersonal and behavioral attributes constitute psychoanalytic cure, how the analysis arrives there is totally unclear. When asked, patients frequently cite the warm personal support they received while in treatment as very significant. Analysts, on the other hand, prefer to focus on the resolution of conflict or the working through of the transference neurosis. Most would assume that the process unfolds gradually, but in fact, it grows in discontinuous steps and leaps. How or why a patient makes a leap at a particular moment in treatment is unknown. Some do so because of a coincidental alignment of external circumstances and others do so because of a fortuitous interaction within the analysis. Cure can occur only when a patient is prepared to let go of the transitional object of the analyst and switch to a more constant object of an independent, flexible, and relatively secure self. Faith is continuously an issue and it also occurs in leaps.

Obviously a most important leap of faith occurs early, in the acceptance of the analyst and the analytic situation which usually involves deprivation and sacrifice on the part of the patient. This is especially difficult for individuals who have paranoid traits or have been physically and/or sexually traumatized. The analysis may then proceed, for some extended length of time before the patient is prepared to make any further leaps. But then, suddenly, heretofore repressed material or erotic feelings consciously withheld are expressed within the transference and a new level of trust is obtained. At some point in virtually all analyses, hateful feelings of the most intense kind erupt within the transference that threaten the very analysis itself. The choice between the negative therapeutic reaction or working through the negative transference and not merely suppressing it or submitting to it, involves a true leap of faith. The next major leap occurs in the transition from the middle phase of analysis to the termination phase. It requires a major leap of faith on the part of the patient no matter how thoroughly s/he had been analyzed up to that point because the commitment to leave analysis is an enormous one. In the termination phase, as the patient finally gives up the object of the analyst, the patient may come to believe that s/he has been faithfully loved even though it has never actually been verbalized directly to her/him.

PHILOSOPHY AND FAITH: UNITY AND DUALITY

Through re-experiencing religious faith, countless individuals (not necessarily in analysis) have found real security even in the face of extreme adversity and peace even at times of personal loss. This is true and has been so for millennia. The active turning to a god image is associated with the re-experience of feelings of security, associated with the earliest moments of object relations.

It has only been in the last century that our Western culture, in the grip of scientific determinism, has swung so completely and unilaterally over to the Hellenistic rational-objective philosophy of truth and away from the Judeo-Christian subjective philosophy of truth. It is worth remembering that so much of our morality and ethical sense has developed from the latter, as technology has flowed from the former. What is also true is that the threat of a loss of faith invariably leads to an inner sense of despair and aggression of some kind, and therefore continues to be of prime importance.

For the ancients, gods, man and society were indivisible and lived in greater harmony with nature. Since those times, mankind has survived with an increasing awareness of self and has struggled to understand and explain his relationship to the world.

Man's representation of God has been a personal one and has paralleled his technological mastery over the world of nature. God has evolved from a simple animal totem representation to a transcendent being who is simultaneously both extraneous and imminent to "creation." Medieval philosophers and theologians since, have contemplated the separate natures of man and God and have tied the relationship of one to the other through faith.

Philosophy made a great leap forward, however, with Spinoza who emerged from his theological studies to conceptualize existence in what is perhaps classic duality terms. In his "Ethics" he described mind and body and physical and mental experiences as parts of one process. They may be perceived in one frame of reference as action and matter "substance" and in the other frame of reference as thoughts and mental "substance." The language applied in one frame of reference cannot be applied in the other and although the entire world may therefore be doubled in this manner, one side cannot exist without the other (Durant, 1961).

Over the next three hundred years philosophy reached its ascendancy and went through what may be called "epistemological wars of first causes." Once God as a concept was dethroned as the originator of all force in the universe, other intellectual theories were necessary to be substituted in its place. Many theories were proposed but generally they divide along the poles of subjective-objective experience and actions. Beginning with Descartes, "I think. Therefore, I am," which is subjectively driven, they covered the spectrum to the systematically objective theories of Kant's "Critique of Pure Reason" (Durant, 1961). One could view consciousness as the central organizing principle with existence being secondary to it. Or, conversely, one could view nature and reality as systematically arranged, with consciousness being only one of its potential creations. The philosophies of Hegel (*Phenomenology of Spirit*), Schopenhauer (*The World as Will and Representation*), Darwin (*Origin of the Species*), and Nietzsche's "Superman" with his will to power, swept through Europe in waves, all in an effort to explain man's fundamental nature (Hamlyn, 1987). God could now be relegated to the position of the indirect originator of "first causes."

The twentieth century began in a breathtaking leap of intellectual creativity in the pursuit of truth. The simultaneous discovery of Einstein's relativistic physics and Freud's unconscious revolutionized age old perceptions of basic physical and mental realities. They in turn gave birth to philosophical movements of the circle of "logical positivists" around Wittgenstein, whose philosophy was restricted to inquiring only about problems that were open to scientific investigation. Simultaneously, the other significant movement was the anti-scientific and metaphysical movement of "existentialism," beginning with Heidegger (Being and Time) and Sartre (Being and Nothingness) (Hamlyn, 1987). The fundamental question for them was why there was anything rather than nothing. Interestingly enough, as the circle turns, now at the end of the twentieth century, astrophysicists, artificial intelligence experts, mathematicians, thermodynamics/physical chemists, and biological theorists are contemplating the same exact questions and they are, perhaps, those most involved with "first causes" and therefore the contemplation of God.

Oddly enough the philosophic father of existentialism was Kierkegaard, who in opposition to the Nietzsche of his day saw truth in a personal relationship in faith (Hamlyn, 1987). Beginning as he did as a seminary student, he found the systematic theories of reasoning, even with the influence of subjective free will, quite limited and falling short of the personal experience of faith. In a world without faith, he argues, man feels that he does not exist. Many years later another existentialist, Jaspers (Truth and Symbol) viewed man as grasping at being in the subject-object polarity with an everlasting need to utilize symbols as ciphers, to a transcendental oneness often referred to as God (Jaspers, 1959). Where Kierkegaard saw man motivated by a personal need for faith, Jaspers saw the need for oneness out of the subject-object polarity.

Object relations theory, therefore, fits neatly with the philosophical dualities of subject-object existence and causation on one hand and the drive to union and oneness on the other. Even language itself, the common symbolic medium for our intellect and comprehension of our experience, is created out of the interplay of internalized object relations. Our explorations of the world, our understanding of our place in it, and our wish to transcend it, no matter how sophisticated, will always be rooted in and simultaneously bounded by the dualities of object relations.

Although modern psychoanalytic theory relies on object relations for its inspiration, it marks a significant departure from classical psychoanalytic theory. Freud's classical system of drives is similar to the first cause theories in philosophy and is related to Fichte's Ich (id) as well as Nietzsche's will to power and the biology inherent in Darwin's *Origin of the Species*. In the classic schema, drives power a biologically bounded neurological system which only later is organized into the mechanistic psychic apparatus of defense and conflict. Only after Freud could the theory be lifted entirely out of the biological frame of reference into the world of object relations. Freud, however, clearly preferred the objective frame of reference for his theory of the personal experience and the scientific method inherent consequently in the neutral observer of phenomena stance in therapy. His considerable efforts in this regard have given rise to a consensually valid system of mind that is ongoing even as it competes with rapid advances in biological brain sciences and neuropsychology.

Ernest Jones has stated that Freud "grew up devoid of any belief in God or immortality and does not appear to have felt a need for it" (Jones, 1956a, p. 465). Even Freud referred to himself as a godless Jew. Nevertheless, he was in fact a man of great morality, ethics and honor. Freud himself cannot explain why he should have been so (Jones, 1956a). Freud was certainly conversant with all Jewish customs and festivals, despite being an atheist. Even though his children were not familiar with Jewish religious traditions (Gay, 1988), throughout his adult life he was certainly preoccupied with religion (Jones, 1956b, 1956c) and maintained a membership in B'nai B'rith. For 30 years he also maintained a very close personal tie to and a strong identification with the Swiss pastor, Oscar Pfister, and in his later years wrote him the following letter after a bout of illness: "Dear Dr. Pfister, After another major operation I am fit for little and uncheerful but, if I had got back some kind of synthesis again by the end of the month–that is what I have been promised– am I to miss the opportunity of seeing my old but by God's grace rejuvenated friend here? Certainly not, I count on it. Cordially yours, Freud" (Meng and Freud, 1963, p. 19).

Its further relevance to the discussion here is also because, with regard to faith, Fromm has rightfully pointed out that "unfortunately the discussion, centered around religion since the days of the

Enlightenment, has been largely concerned with affirmation or negation of certain human attitudes" (Fromm, 1950, p. 133). "Do you believe in God?" has been the crucial question of religionists, and the denial of God has been the position chosen by those fighting the church. But it is easy to see that many who profess the belief in God are in their human attitude idol worshipers filled with hate and men without faith while some of the most ardent "atheists" devoting their lives to the betterment of mankind, to deeds of brotherliness and love, have exhibited faith and a profoundly religious attitude (Fromm 1950).

Freud, it would seem, was an example of such a man and it is reasonable to conclude that a part of his motivation in his constant creative struggle and his preoccupation with Moses was, among other things, an effort to maintain a close identification with and a tie to the faith of his father.

CONCLUSION

This short paper can do little justice to the subject of psychoanalysis and faith, and is intended only as a beginning. First, this review should not be understood as a blanket endorsement of theism or religion (particularly that of a submissive, compulsive and ritualistic type), but clearly psychoanalysis now nearly 100 years after its inception needs to address the centrality of faith in development and growth instead of disregarding its importance to our patients. Insofar as faith is an outgrowth of early development, it must be fundamental to self and as a uniquely human experience deserves as much attention in our analytic work as other concepts ordinarily receive. Both psychoanalysts and theologians have equal claims upon the area of faith and probably have much to say to each other. Both seek truth and in so doing strive for the highest in human attainment. Both also seek to understand aggression and the means to prevent its unwarranted expression.

Second, we need to recognize that from the first contact until the last session, faith is a central issue and is always being remodelled. It does not proceed smoothly or continuously but in "leaps" that are discontinuous and unpredictable. Further investigation is necessary to determine why in analysis some individuals are prepared to make those leaps of faith and eventually move on to termination while others are fixated and therefore remain alienated, distrustful, and insecure.

Third, it would appear that successful psychoanalytic technique involves not two, but three, important components: (1) the examination of unconscious drives and internal object relations and the conflicts contained within them; (2) the experience of the dyadic relationship and the clarification of the distortions within the transference; and (3) the recognition of the critical importance of a working through process that not only expands the intellectual awareness but also consolidates the gains in trust as it prepares the patient for further leaps of faith to a progressively more flexible and more truthful self, a self that can tolerate loss without excessive anxiety or aggression.

Without a recognition of the importance of faith in the third component, we create highly intellectualized but otherwise persistently anxious analytic dependents. Only with the attainment of the balanced and co-equal pair of awareness and faith can we say that we have effected cure in our patients.

REFERENCES

Aron, L. Free Association and Changing Models of Mind. *Journal of the American Academy of Psychoanalysis* 18:439-459, 1990.

Balint, M. *The Basic Fault: Therapeutic Aspects of Regression.* New York: Brunner/Mazel, 1968.

Buber, M. *Two Types of Faith.* New York: Macmillan Publishing Company, 1951.

Buber, M. *The Way of Man: According to the Teaching of Hasidism.* New Jersey: Citadel Press, 1966.

Danielian, J., Lister, E. The Negative Therapeutic Reaction: The Uses of Negation. *Journal of the American Academy of Psychoanalysis* 16:431-450, 1988.

Durant, W. *The Story of Philosophy.* New York: Pocket Books, 1961.

Eigen, M. The Area of Faith in Winnicott, Lacan and Bion. *International Journal of Psychoanalysis* 62:418, 1981.

Eigen, M. Toward Bion's Staring Point: Between Catastrophe and Faith. *International Journal of Psychoanalysis* 66:321-330, 1985.

Freud, S. *The Future of an Illusion,* in Standard Edition 21, 1961.

Fromm, E. *Psychoanalysis and Religion.* Connecticut: Yale University Press, 1950.

Gay, P. *Freud: A Life for Our Time.* London: W.W. Norton & Co., 1988.

Gill, M. *Theory and Technique,* Vol I. Analysis of Transference. Connecticut: International University Press, 1982.

Hamlyn, D.W. *A History of Western Philosophy.* London: Pelican Books, 1987.

Jackel, M.M. Transference and Psychotherapy. *Psychoanalysis Quarterly* 40:43-58, 1966.

Jaspers, K. *Truth and Symbol.* New York: Twayne Publishers, 1959.

Jones, E. *Sigmund Freud:* Letter to J.J. Putnam, 8 July 1915, Vol. 2. London: Hogorth Press, 1956a.

Jones, E. *Sigmund Freud,* Vol 3. London: Hogorth Press, 1956b.

Jones, E. *Sigmund Freud,* Vol 7. London: Hogorth Press, 1956c.

Kernberg, O. *Internal World and External Reality.* New York: Aronson, 1980.

Langs, R. *Truth Therapy/Lie Therapy in Classics in Psychoanalytic Technique.* Edited by Langs, R. New York: Aronson, pp. 499-515, 1981.

Mahler, M.S., Pine, F., Bergman, A. *The Psychological Birth of the Human Infant.* New York: Basic Books, 1975.

Mann, J. Clinical and Theoretical Aspects of Religious Belief. *Journal of the Am Psychoanalytic Association* 12:160-170, 1962.

Meng, H., Freud, E. (eds). *Psychoanalysis and Faith: The Letters of Sigmund Freud and Oskar Pfister.* New York: Basic Books, 1963.

Ogden, T.H. The Concept of Internal Object Relations. *International Journal Psychoanalysis* 64:227-241, 1984.

Tarachow, S. *An Introduction to Psychotherapy.* New York: International University Press, 1963.

Tuttman, S. Exploring the Analyst's Treatment Stance in Current Psychoanalytic Practice. *Journal of the American Academy of Psychoanalysis* 15:29-37, 1987.

Wallerstein, R. One Psychoanalysis or many? *International Journal of Psychoanalysis* 36:3-30, 1988.

Response to
"The Role of Faith in Mental Healing: Psychoanalysis and Faith"

This chapter puts questions of faith squarely within the practice of psychoanalysis. Dr. Bronheim states that "faith as a uniquely human experience is frequently encountered in psychoanalytic practice, and faith overlaps with psychoanalysis in bringing about cure." Though Dr. Bronheim's perspective is not my perspective, I am an admirer of his perspective. My perspective is from a faith community, as one who hears both the faith questions and the psychological struggles of my parishioners.

At this hour last Wednesday, I stood in front of 300 people who had come to a funeral service looking for comfort and reassurance in their grief for the loss of a 30-year-old man who had died of colon cancer. As in crucial sessions of analysis, what is said at an occasion like that must be true, responsive and based ultimately on a belief in something greater than the dynamics of speaker to hearer.

Another piece of this story is important. Two days before the funeral, both parents said, "Toby, this sucks." I thought about that for a week. What were they saying? As their pastor, which I had been in the past, they would never have said that to me, but under these circumstances both of them individually said the same thing. I think what they were saying is that they were able, as faithful people with death still fresh in their eyes, to begin to address their anger and their hurt at the loss of a precious son. In both cases anger was

[Haworth co-indexing entry note]: *"Response* to "The Role of Faith in Mental Healing: Psychoanalysis and Faith.""* Gould, The Reverend Toby. Co-published simultaneously in the *Journal of Religion in Disability & Rehabilitation* (The Haworth Press, Inc.) Vol. 1, No. 2, 1994, pp. 19-21; and: *Pastoral Care of the Mentally Disabled: Advancing Care of the Whole Person* (ed: Sally K. Severino, and The Reverend Richard Liew) The Haworth Press, Inc., 1994, pp. 19-21. Multiple copies of this article/chapter may be purchased from The Haworth Document Delivery Center [1-800-3-HAWORTH; 9:00 a.m. - 5:00 p.m. (EST)].

focused, for the moment at least, not on their loss but aimed at a "capricious or uncaring deity." Within minutes, those same parents sat down around their kitchen table, and together we planned the funeral service for their son. It was clear that day and during the funeral that people were looking to their faith for comfort and for strength. Certainly, this is one area of common ground.

While I cannot argue with Dr. Bronheim's assertion that "in the vast psychiatric literature on loss and grief there is little discussion on the appearance of faith," the converse of that is not true. From Job to Jesus to Buddha, religious leaders have addressed feelings of grief face-on. The field of pastoral counseling which brings us here today has much to say on the subject of grief, from the understanding of both faith and psychology. Perhaps analysts could learn from pastoral counselors that a well-grounded faith can aid in the process of moving through the stages of grief. A dialogue between analysts and faith communities might need to limit those faith communities to ones sharing similar traditions. Terravodic Buddhists and Shiite Moslems, both coming from ancient faith communities, share almost nothing in common in term of history or beliefs. While Christian Fundamentalists and Unitarians share a biblical history, on good days, these groups could hardly agree on one point of doctrine. In fact, Unitarians don't always accept doctrine as a category. Within so-called mainstream Protestant churches, there is a variety of beliefs, practices and customs which are profound enough to be recognized as distinct in a discussion with those outside that faith community, e.g., psychoanalysts.

Dr. Bronheim's paper aims for universal conclusions, courtesy of 20th century philosophy for the most part, while the major religions of the world tend to draw their strength from their particularities. If there is to be a true dialogue between psychoanalysis and the faith community, this question needs to be answered: Are practitioners of psychoanalysis prepared to deal with faith questions, not only in terms of psychodynamics but also within the notion that the system of belief held by the patient or client is something beyond delusion or fantasy? If Freud did write that sometimes a cigar is indeed a cigar, my personal belief structure states that sometimes God is, in fact, God. That is, God is not only the image of my belief, but the object of my belief, and no amount of personal insight or philosophical speculation can get around that objective category. In the words of Phillip Watson, who taught me theology, sometimes at least, let God be God.

I would like very much to see pastoral counselors and theologians wrestle with the concept set forth by Dr. Bronheim: "Faith is the essential emotional state that enables a positive inner image of the object to be sustained irrespective of either satisfaction or dissatisfaction, and may undergo remodeling throughout the life cycle." To me, that statement comes close to saying that God, as the object of faith, is an independent actor. It posits the possibility of God. Yet Dr. Bronheim drags us through the American ego-psychology school and British object-relations school going at faith with every blunt object at their command. I would take from the quotes, that the object of their rage is not faith, but God. From neurotically anxious Catholics to inflamed members of the Hasidim, we are taken through the fixations and permutations of the psychologically and religiously troubled.

There is a place for Protestant clergy in the diagnostic tools of analysis. The business of psychoanalysis has been to deal with the presenting and underlying problems of patients who come for help. I would hope that the field could look to the securing of healthy faith as a goal, rather than just the elimination of an unhealthy faith as cure. Dr. Bronheim mentioned Martin Buber as a modern practitioner of faith who happens to use story idioms to reach the mind, heart and soul of those who are curious and questing for a mature faith. I would suggest that Paul Tillich, Abraham Heschel, Paul Tournier, Harold Kushner, and Frederick Buechner could be added to the list of those who take psychological and theological categories seriously.

The Reverend Toby Gould, MDiv

Response to
"The Role of Faith in Mental Healing: Psychoanalysis and Faith"

While wondering about what to say in response to Dr. Bronheim's multifaceted paper, I asked my wife "Well, what do you think about psychiatry and faith?" She said, "When I was a girl growing up in a small town in California, attending an Episcopalian Sunday school, I used to ask, when they told us Bible stories, 'How do you know this is true? Maybe it's just an interesting story. Maybe there's a lesson in it for us, but how do you know it's true?' I said it so many times that I got to be a real pain-in-the-neck for the Sunday school teacher. She finally sent me home with a note to my parents instructing them to take me to a psychiatrist." So there's no doubt there's a deep connection between psychiatry and faith.

Dr. Bronheim's talk and paper highlighted two very important views; one is the conceptualization of faith in terms of object-relations. The second is the process of therapy as an act of faith. I am going to comment on the second. When I read Dr. Bronheim's paper, I was inspired to think about my own experiences as a therapist and what role faith plays in the therapies that I conduct. I would broaden Dr. Bronheim's notion of the role of faith in psychoanalysis to all healing relationships. I thought of the clinical and technical term, "placebo effect," which exerts a profound and powerful influence on outcomes in all of medicine. It refers to the power of faith in the treatment or in the doctor to boost the therapeutic result. That's

[Haworth co-indexing entry note]: *"Response* to "The Role of Faith in Mental Healing: Psychoanalysis and Faith." " Polan, H. Jonathan. Co-published simultaneously in the *Journal of Religion in Disability & Rehabilitation* (The Haworth Press, Inc.) Vol. 1, No. 2, 1994, pp. 23-25; and: *Pastoral Care of the Mentally Disabled: Advancing Care of the Whole Person* (ed: Sally K. Severino, and The Reverend Richard Liew) The Haworth Press, Inc., 1994, pp. 23-25. Multiple copies of this article/chapter may be purchased from The Haworth Document Delivery Center [1-800-3-HAWORTH; 9:00 a.m. - 5:00 p.m. (EST)].

23

why new medications must be tested against placebo-controlled groups.

But the patient's faith in the doctor or the therapist is not the only kind of faith important in therapy. The therapist must also have faith in the patient. I think it was Hans Loewald who said that the essential role of the therapist is to be the "guardian of the patient's potential." That, in essence, requires faith in the patient. Although a patient's current behaviors may be self-defeating, the therapist must create his or her own mental image of this person becoming a fulfilled, responsible person. The therapist must believe in that image and guard its integrity through possibly long periods of acting out on the part of the patient.

Patients will ask, "Don't you trust me?" Their question, "Don't you trust me?" is as important to them as their question, "Can I trust you?" Maybe some of you have patients for whom, at some point in therapy, "Don't you trust me?" seems to be the predominant with which you struggle. Patients might make suicide gestures and when you advise that they refrain from alcohol or that they call you, they ask "Don't you trust me?" As therapist you have to communicate to such patients that, while you don't trust their current behavior, on another level, a deeper level of the relationship, you have faith in them.

Patients also must have faith in being themselves. That is another act of faith, and an important one. In a sense, then, there is a triangular faith system in psychotherapy: the patient-therapist (the patient has to have faith in the therapist), the therapist-patient (the therapist has to have faith in the patient), and the patient-him/herself. Perhaps not all of these faith relationships, or legs of the triangle, have to be equally active simultaneously, but at least one of them has to be active at all times. Otherwise, the therapy can come to a stop and the therapeutic enterprise may fail. Let me give two vignettes from patients in my practice to illustrate these thoughts. In the first, the patient's faith in himself saved the therapy, and in the second, my faith in the patient saved the therapy.

Mr. S., a man in his forties, came to me shortly after having started his own business. He had not been successful at his old job, but he thought having escaped his overwhelming boss, he might do better on his own. He described his father as an extremely domineering, highly competitive, self-centered, very successful businessman whom he resented but wanted to emulate. I have to confess that

I did not visualize this man as a successful salesman. His specific complaint, which he wanted me to work on right away, was that he was so anxious when he went to call on potential customers, he couldn't get to the point of closing the sale. And instead of making several sales calls a day, he was making one. In an awkward effort to relieve his very high anxiety, I said, "Maybe you're just not cut out to be a salesman." I have learned that this patient does not usually hear what I say until I have said it five or six times. So, luckily he did not process my statement. I suspect he does not remember I said that to him and, as it turns out, he is a talented salesman, clearly on his way to becoming an independent businessman with a good deal of potential. I would say that it was his faith in himself which saved the therapy.

Ms. B., an unmarried woman in her thirties, was referred to me after a psychiatric hospitalization for a near-fatal suicide attempt by overdose. She had a long history of alcoholism and was drinking the night of the overdose. She established a very strong attachment to me right away, and worked well in therapy until I went on vacation. Two weeks prior to my vacation she started to skip appointments and not answer her phone. When I did reach her, it seemed to me she was intoxicated, which she denied. She didn't show up for her last appointment before my vacation. Knowing she was in her high-rise apartment, I called her, but there was no answer. I went to her apartment, had the super let me in, and found her with liquor in the apartment. Clearly she was terrified of and enraged at my going on vacation, but she did not say that; instead, she vented her feelings at me for invading her privacy and treating her like a child. She refused to come with me to my office, and refused to make an appointment to see my covering doctor. I had to decide whether to have her taken to the hospital to be admitted against her will. She insisted she was not going to harm herself. I then made one of the most difficult decisions of my career. Something deep within me told me to leave her alone. I, of course, was worried about her throughout my vacation. On my return I found that she had checked into the hospital for detox right after I left. Two years later, still in therapy, she's doing extremely well. By following my instincts, I took a risk, but placed my faith in her.

H. Jonathan Polan, MD

The Role of Mental Health
in Spiritual Growth

The Reverend Walter J. Smith, SJ, PhD

My task is to reflect with you on the relationship between mental health and spiritual growth. The very pairing of these two topics could excite both psychologists and theologians, either of whom might wish to argue that no significant relationship exists between the two concepts. Conclusions about their mutual antagonism or compatibility depend, of course, on prior assumptions one makes about both components of the relationship.

As both priest and clinical psychologist, as believer and skeptic, I am caught professionally in the middle of this confrontation, navigating the perilous waters between Scylla and Charybdis. However, I feel assured to explore this issue in this conference setting, since our purpose is precisely to discover points of mutuality between mental health and spirituality.

Among mental health practitioners and theorists, spirituality and spiritual growth are terms burdened by stereotype and negative association. Rarely would one expect to find these issues paired with a discussion of positive mental health. If anything, spirituality and religion have been considered by some psychiatrists and psychologists to be among the root causes of neuroses and mental illness.

One of the expressed purposes of this symposium is to "mend the

[Haworth co-indexing entry note]: "The Role of Mental Health in Spiritual Growth." Smith, The Reverend Walter J., SJ. Co-published simultaneously in the *Journal of Religion in Disability & Rehabilitation* (The Haworth Press, Inc.) Vol. 1, No. 2, 1994, pp. 27-40; and: *Pastoral Care of the Mentally Disabled: Advancing Care of the Whole Person* (ed: Sally K. Severino, and The Reverend Richard Liew) The Haworth Press, Inc., 1994, pp. 27-40. Multiple copies of this article/chapter may be purchased from The Haworth Document Delivery Center [1-800-3-HAWORTH; 9:00 a.m. - 5:00 p.m. (EST)].

mind," to narrow the chasm that separates issues which we assert are complementary and reciprocally beneficial. Mental health, as we shall view it throughout the course of this discussion, is integral to spiritual growth, and a mature spirituality can promote and help maintain a person's mental health.

THEORETICAL ANTECEDENTS

Without realizing it at the time, I suspect the foundations for this address were established more than thirty years ago when I was a university student in Boston and attended a lecture by Abraham Maslow at Brandeis University where he was the first chairman of the Department of Psychology. The essence of his presentation was later summarized in a paper and published in the inaugural issues of the *Journal of Humanistic Psychology* (Maslow, 1961).

Dr. Maslow was strongly opposed to defining psychological health simply in terms of adjustment to reality, society, and other people. He vigorously argued against defining a healthy person in terms of his or her abilities to master the environment; to be capable, adequate, effective, and competent in relation to it; to do a good job, to be successful in a task—definitions of mental health that were current at that time, and which continue to figure into current discussions.

One reason I recall Maslow's presentation with such clarity is that it was optimistic, almost utopian in its perspective of the human person. Coming from psychoanalytic training as I did, Maslow's perspective was fresh and engaging. For all that I owe to Freud's thought and method, I have always been disquieted by what I perceived as a growing despair in Freud's view of the human person, culminating in a view that sees civilization as a veneer incapable of ever really doing much to counteract the human person's destructive instincts.

Maslow avowed that the healthy person is characterized by an ability to transcend other people's opinions. We have to remember, Maslow was unfolding this understanding in the 1950s and 1960s, long before the contemporary liberation movements and dramatic social changes that have shaped the past three decades of our American society.

Maslow presented mental health in terms of self-mastery, of an ability to think and act autonomously, in terms of an ability to look within the self for guiding values and rules to live by. "Only by such a differentiation can we leave a theoretical place for meditation, contemplation, and for all other forms of going into the self, of turning away from the outer world in order to listen to the inner voices" (Maslow 1961, p. 1).

Maslow had a particular interest in the change in understanding among mental health theorists and practitioners concerning the role of the unconscious, of primary process and of the mythological and poetic. "Because the roots of ill health were found in the unconscious, it has been our tendency to think of the unconscious as bad, evil, crazy, dirty, or dangerous and to think of the primary processes as distorting the truth. But now that we have found these depths to be also the source of creativeness, of art, of love, of humor, and play, and even of certain kinds of truth and knowledge, we can begin to speak of a healthy unconscious, of healthy regressions. And especially, we can begin to value primary process cognition and archaic or mythological thinking instead of considering them to be pathological.

We can now go into primary process cognitions for certain kinds of knowledge, not only about the self but also about the world, to which secondary processes are blind. These primary processes are part of the normal or healthy human nature and must be included in any comprehensive theory of human nature" (Maslow, 1961, p. 1).

It is now, many years later, that I am drawn to revisit this event of my university education, and the formative influence that this son of Russian Jewish immigrants has had on my understanding of the relationship between mental health and spirituality. It is only now that I have come to appreciate that Maslow was as much an ethicist as a humanistic psychologist; he would have been at home in this conference exploring the care of the whole person. He searched to uncover a set of principles for living a human life that could be described as morally good. Psychology was a tool to make that discovery possible.

Isn't this after all what Joseph Campbell means when he says, "People say what we're all seeking is a meaning for life. I don't think that's what we're really seeking. I think what we're seeking is an experience of being alive, so that our life experiences on the purely physical plane will have resonances within our own innermost being and reality, so that we actually feel the rapture of being alive. That's what it's finally about, and that's what these clues help us to find within ourselves" (Campbell, 1988, p. 5).

It is not my desire to reintroduce into our discussion today a false dualism that divorces body from spirit, mental health from spirituality. We all know the efforts of the past which proceeded on an assumption that the spiritual person, purified of all material concerns, strives to attain the pure realm of the soul and the spirit. Nor do I want to suggest a reduction of spirituality to the purely psychological or sociological. Mental health and spirituality are distinct but related aspects of human development. Our concern today is to explore the interrelationships.

GOALS

I would like to address the following objectives: building on a formulation of personality dynamics and mental health rooted in humanistic psychological theory, I would like to consider the implications for spiritual growth; reciprocally, I would like to consider the potential in spirituality both for health and healing. To achieve these objectives, I shall present a case study of a thirty-year-old man with HIV disease, who was referred for psychological counseling. As his mental health needs were addressed systematically in the course of treatment, spiritual growth and religious practice became an unanticipated focus of his expressed concerns. The case, which extended in treatment for 26 months until his death in 1990, will help to exemplify some of the observations I offer in the first part of this presentation.

SPIRITUAL GROWTH

Spirituality is the human capacity to go beyond ourselves in the search for truth and knowledge, in loving relationships and in a freedom to commit ourselves to other persons and to human tasks.

What actualizes this capacity? How is it expressed? How does this aspect of the human personality develop? These are some of the questions psychology and religion seek to investigate.

We are not simply viewing another trend when we note the renaissance of popular interest in spirituality. Spirituality is an essential component of the human personality. To deny the presence of a spiritual dimension is to introduce a schism into the human person.

One way of conceptualizing mental health is as a process that tries to embrace the 'spiritual' component, which somehow has been split apart from the 'material' component. Used in this sense, spirituality is a comprehensive term, defining philosophical and psychological as well as religious variables. In fact, spirituality or spiritual growth is a more accessible term precisely because it is so inclusive. We have noted in our professional practice numerous individuals who claim no 'religious' affiliation, yet who speak with comfort about the 'spiritual' component in their lives.

Returning again to Joseph Campbell, we find another way in which this spiritual dimension is described and accessed: "There has to be a training to help you open your ears so that you can begin to hear metaphorically instead of concretely. Freud and Jung both felt that myth is grounded in the unconscious. Anyone writing a creative work knows that you open, you yield yourself and the book talks to you and builds itself. To a certain extent, you become the carrier of something that is given to you from what have been called the Muses—or, in biblical language, God.

This is no fancy, it is a fact. Since the inspiration comes from the unconscious, and since the unconscious minds of the people of any small society have much in common, what the shaman or seer brings forth is something that is waiting to be brought forth in everyone. So when one hears the seer's story, one responds, 'Aha! This is my story. This is something I have always wanted to say but wasn't able to say.' There has to be a dialogue, an interaction between the seer and the community. . . . The folk tale is for entertainment; the myth is for spiritual instruction" (Campbell, 1988, pp. 58-59).

It is my assumption that all of life can function like the shaman or seer's story, can be a means for engaging the spiritual dimension, can promote becoming whole, or expressed in religious language, for becoming "holy." Let us look concretely at how these relations are played out in human life.

MENTAL HEALTH: THE HUMANISTIC VIEW

One of the more attractive aspects of viewing mental health within a humanistic perspective is its optimism. It is a view of the human person that is compatible with the Judeo-Christian religious tradition.

In the book of Genesis, when God reviews the work of creation, including the fashioning of man and woman, we read the refrain, "And God looked at everything God had made, and found it very good" (Genesis 1:31). The tradition also notes that God gave man and woman dominion over the created order, to steward these resources in order that they might achieve the full potential for which they were created. So, too, mental health stresses the roles each individual's unique potential and experiences play in shaping his or her own existence.

Contrasted with a Freudian perception of human nature as self-interested, despite the veneer of civilization, the humanistic perspective is both positive and constructive, assuming that at the root of human nature one discovers goodness. This spiritual force, if released and expressed, is meant to help the individual achieve his or her full potential as person.

These assumptions about the human person cast a number of issues in a different light. If we did not begin with assumptions that our natural instincts are selfish and acquisitive, we might not be so distrustful of our impulses, desires, and feelings as Freud suggests.

Another aspect of a humanistic definition of mental health is its proactive approach. Human persons are seen as self-determining. Expressed in philosophical terms, human persons are "oriented to the good." In a sense, humans are imprinted to act out of this "goodness" as long as their essential needs are satisfied.

Human persons are always becoming, always challenged to further possibilities for growth. These possibilities precipitate crises that require choices in directing growth. In this sense crises can be seen as helpful in as much as they open possibilities for individual growth.

THE INTERPLAY BETWEEN MENTAL HEALTH
AND SPIRITUALITY:
THE CASE OF MATTHEW

At the outset I indicated that I would like to pursue this discussion by considering a case that unexpectedly placed the relationship between mental health and spirituality in bold relief.

While serving as academic dean of a theological school in Cambridge, Massachusetts, I volunteered several hours of professional service each week to public welfare clients of the Adult AIDS Unit at The Boston City Hospital. Matthew, recently diagnosed as HIV positive and asymptomatic, was referred by his physician for counseling.

Matthew was the youngest in a family of 12 children. Both of his parents were chronic alcoholics, with erratic histories of recovery and relapse. Matt left home when he was 14 years of age and moved to the West Coast where he survived through prostitution, selling drugs, and by involvement in other illicit activities.

In his late adolescence, he met an older man with whom he lived for almost six years in return for sexual favors. After living almost 15 years away from his family of origin, Matt found his way back to his place of birth and began to address his addictions through involvement in Alcoholics Anonymous. At the suggestion of his sponsor, he was tested for HIV and was reported to be positive.

After Matt received the results of the antibody test, he was referred to a hospital-based support group, facilitated by a social worker experienced in working with HIV clients. After learning of his seropositive status, neither AA nor the support group was successful in addressing the anxieties, fears, and night tremors that Matthew reported to his physician. He was also quite explosive in the clinic, often acting out his aggression in hostile and verbally abusive ways toward the medical and nursing staff. Because of his attempts to remain drug-free, he was resistant to the suggestion of anxiolytic medication to help him manage his feelings. The medical team judged that individual counseling might offer some relief, which other interventions were not able to achieve.

Matt was quite willing to accept an offer of individual counseling, since he reported so much subjective pain and found much of daily living to be stressful. He reported that he often felt as if he were "losing it," which meant he felt out of control. He was frightened, fearful that he would start to drink again, smoke dope, and use cocaine as a way of dulling the pain he was experiencing. Counseling represented a possible solution to his problems. His seropositive status was indeed a concern, but it did not command the same attention as the anxious feelings about which he spoke so freely.

Although Matthew had little formal education beyond junior high school, he was very intelligent and highly verbal. He was also street-smart and cunning. It was this natural and acquired knowledge that insured his survival through his adolescent and young adult years. He read people and situations with remarkable accuracy.

After almost three months of weekly sessions which focused on management of problems of daily living, decision-making, and impulse control, he announced at the beginning of one session that he was finally ready to begin therapy. As he unpacked this declaration, he said that it had taken him this long to be convinced that the therapist was trustworthy. Matt said: "My whole life has been a story of survival. Every man I've ever known wanted something from me—booze, drugs, money, my body. I've sat here week after week trying to figure out what's in this for you. You don't take any money; I wondered when the other shoe would drop, when your real motive would become clear. This past week, I finally thought, maybe there are some people in the world who really care. I figure that I have to take a chance that you're one of those kind of people. My life is out of order, and you're the only person right now who says you will stand by me and help me sort it out. Coming here on the bus today I thought, "You've really got to give him the benefit of the doubt—it's your last chance!"

For the first four months Matt had been asymptomatic; then he developed Kaposi lesions on his leg, which warranted a definitive diagnosis of AIDS. He maintained regular counseling contact throughout the final 15 months of his battle with several HIV-related illnesses, despite the fact that treatments were debilitating and some required hospitalizations.

The psychotherapy relationship provided Matthew a place to sort out his feelings and order his thinking; it was a safe environment in which he explored his options, where he formulated and tested his decisions. Psychotherapy was not a mysterious or esoteric experience for this perceptive and astute young man; it was a place in which his dreams and fantasies, his feelings and desires, his motivation and understanding could unfold and be processed.

As I noted above, Matthew found this experience so beneficial that he rarely missed an appointment, even when his health deteriorated and made transportation difficult. There were times when he left a hospital or a difficult clinical procedure like a bronchoscopy and came directly to the therapist's office for a session. And he was never unprepared.

During his treatment, he reviewed his family history, his adolescence and young adult experiences, his struggles with drugs, and the full range of his relationships. He talked honestly about HIV disease, his approach to its treatment and his anticipated death. He set definite goals and invited help in achieving these objectives. For example, he investigated how he might earn a high school equivalency diploma, although he never realized this goal. The most significant goal was to establish an independent residence for himself. With the help of a local AIDS Action Committee, he was able to rent and furnish a small apartment in a low-income housing complex and to live in this apartment during the final seven months of his life.

As treatment progressed, despite the increasing demands placed on him by his HIV-related illnesses and their medical treatments, Matt's mental health improved steadily. The presenting symptoms of anxiety, sleep disturbance, and paranoia abated, and he began to feel more competent in a wide array of relationships and tasks. The anxious feelings began to dissipate gradually. He became more serene and less prone to panic. He re-established relationships with many members of his family and was able to live with the limits imposed on him by his family members' addictions and other dysfunctional behaviors.

He reported that he slept better, and the dream sequences he recounted were notably less violent than those described earlier in his treatment. He was able to use materials he learned from his dreams, and began to see positive aspects of his personality that until this time remained hidden from him. His overall affect was more positive and his behavior toward the medical staff who managed his physical care was remarkably more cooperative and appreciative. He took greater responsibility for his life and enjoyed the independence that flowed from many of his decisions.

As his overall mental health improved steadily, he experienced a religious reawakening, which he began to explore in the psychotherapeutic context. These themes and experiences were expressed not only in his images and speech, but also in his dreams and fantasies. They were the subject of initiatives he was exploring in terms of religious practice and ritual. At a point when his therapy was concluding, what he began seeking from his therapist was more spiritual direction than psychological counseling.

Because both his primary physician and his therapist were Roman Catholic priests–a fact he knew from the outset of his relationship with them–he felt quite comfortable using "therapy time" to help him sort out some of his spiritual experiences. His physician noted that these themes frequently surfaced in his conversations with Matthew, a phenomenon not present earlier in their relationship.

For the psychotherapist, it was clear that exploring these spiritual issues was as important to Matthew's overall healthy functioning as anything else that had been part of the therapeutic relationship. It became apparent that the antecedent work addressing basic mental health concerns, and notable progress Matthew made on this frontier, facilitated the surfacing of spiritual issues in Matthew's consciousness in ways that demanded attention and expression.

As a child, Matthew had been baptized in the Roman Catholic faith but he had not been exposed to either formal religious education or practice. For example, he never received the sacraments of penance, Eucharist, or confirmation. He did not learn formal prayers, nor did he attend Mass.

Among the ways in which spiritual direction assisted him was to supply basic religious education, which prepared him to seek full incorporation into the Church of his youth. He wanted to learn how to pray, and responded well to traditional devotional practices. He used a small book of prayers that he received on the occasion of his first communion, and these prayers brought him much consolation.

His faith-life was simple and yet strong. He was drawn to reading the Scriptures and was naturally able to meditate and pray with these texts. As the spiritual dimension developed, he felt increasingly more confident of his abilities to manage all aspects of his life and illness. It was almost as if the success of the therapeutic relationships he had with both physician and psychologist had opened a path of an understanding relationship to God. On several different occasions he explicitly addressed this similarity. The common thread was trust and confidence that another person cares.

His several serious illnesses disposed him to direct and comfortable discussions about death. In the latter part of the relationship, death was always situated in the language of returning to God. These conversations were thoughtful and uncovered a primitive but strong faith. He drew enormous comfort from the notion of "communion of saints." For the first time in his life, he was relating to healthy notions of community and family. When he thought about his own death, he imagined it in terms of a reunion with Jesus and Mary, and with many of the saints whom he was meeting through reading brief accounts of their lives.

A year before his death he received the sacraments of penance, confirmation, and the anointing of the sick. He received Holy Communion at a Eucharistic celebration attended by many members of his family, including both his parents, three siblings, nephews and nieces, as well as his physician, his AA sponsor, and others in his support team. The family organized itself sufficiently well for this milestone occasion that it prepared and hosted a party following the small, private celebration of Matthew's confirmation and first communion.

During his final year of life, he met another person with HIV who was 15 years his senior. They became close friends and Matthew assumed the role of primary care provider for this other person who, at the time they met, was considerably more advanced with AIDS. Matthew used his own counseling as a way to monitor his relationship, as well as to develop strategies to resolve conflicts that arose. Because independence and autonomy were basic needs, he often evaluated his experiences in light of these issues, making them the litmus test of his mental health and functioning.

Before Matthew died in June, 1990, he received anointing and communion one final time. In his last conversation with his counselor before his death, he summarized what this relationship had meant to him. He returned to the theme that had been the turning point of his treatment. Noting that in his whole life he had never known a relationship with another man where there had not been a sexual, exploitative, manipulative, or abusive agenda, he was doubtful that anyone could love another "unconditionally," to borrow an expression from Carl Rogers. Matthew confessed that for a long time he wondered why anyone would do so much for him without expecting something in return. He said that this was decisive in his coming to understand the relationship between himself and God.

In his mind, this was the pivotal turning point, the time when he began to trust confidently, to hope enthusiastically and to accept being loved without fear of abandonment. Just short of his thirty-second birthday, Matthew died. His final words to me, spoken in a labored whisper, were these: "Looking back on my life, I many times asked myself why God would send someone like you into my life at this time. Now I know the answer. God does love me and sent me an angel to bring me home. You've been that angel, and I want you to know how much this has meant to me. When the days were the darkest, you were always there. You helped me through some rough times. You said you would stay with me to the end, and you have. Thank you my friend. I love you."

Before I conclude, let me offer a few observations on this case by way of discussion. All of us know that the practice of psychotherapy in the treatment of mental disorders requires the continual modification of the practitioner's system or methodology in accordance with the needs and problems of each individual patient. The result, of course, is that the underlying personality theory to which the practitioner subscribes is altered or changed as a result of his/her practice.

In my own approach to the therapeutic process, I have always guarded the hierarchic valuing of the care for persons over the care for theories. Each of the major systems of personality and psychotherapy has made it's own contribution to a body of knowledge about how to assist persons with mental afflictions. Few of these theories or approaches have tapped the potential for healing and health in spirituality.

Freud suggested that religion is based on unconscious, primitive, and irrational psychic processes; he thought that some religious beliefs are a form of schizophrenia and some practices a form of obsessive-compulsive psychoneuroses, different from the psychiatric syndromes only in that they are socially accepted. Few theorists and practitioners have ventured to consider the interrelationship of spirituality and mental health.

In this paper I have not dismissed this critique of spirituality and religious practice simply because I do not like this formulation. However, in the case I have presented, I have observed how a psychotherapeutic process undertaken to address a number of psychological disturbances opened a whole wealth of therapeutic resources that can be best labelled "spiritual." Arieti (1967) and others have countered Freud's arguments, and have affirmed the potential for health and healing that exists in the resources of spirituality and religion.

Matthew's case is but one clinical example of the way in which an accepting, supportive, and encouraging relationship not only helped to reduce stress symptoms, but it also helped the patient access what Maslow described as the inner place "for meditation, contemplation, and for all other forms of going into the self . . . "

If there was any significant reorganization taking place in Matthew's life in the final 26 months in which we worked together, it was in this arena of the spirit. Psychotherapy, as we all appreciate, does not always take place consciously; many of its helpful effects are gradual, unconscious, almost imperceptible. They are achieved as the balance is altered in a person's life between disturbed elements and constructive ones.

What we observed in Matthew's case was what happened as his fears, anger, resentment, and guilt were addressed. The spiritual resources were uncovered, identified, affirmed, and utilized productively in the service of health and healing. In this remarkable case, the relationship with the therapist proved vital not only for improvements in the areas of psychological functioning, but equally as important, in the area of spiritual awakening and growth through a relationship with his caregivers that was rooted in trust and commitment, Matthew experienced the forces within himself that helped him realign his personality in the direction of health. Psychotherapy was not a replacement for spirituality; and vice versa, spirituality is not a replacement for psychotherapy. Both have a place in the comprehensive care of persons–even for those for whom there is not nor has there ever been a religious identification.

With your indulgence, I would like to conclude with a reference to selected verses from Psalm 91, which in its ancient expression, seeks to mend the mind and mind the soul:

> Say to the Lord, 'My refuge and my fortress,
>   my God in whom I trust.'
> For God will rescue you from the snare of the fowler, from the
>   destroying pestilence.
> With pinions he will cover you, and under his wings you shall
>   take refuge;
> God's faithfulness is a buckler and a shield. You shall not fear
>   the terror of the night nor the arrow that flies by day;
> Not the pestilence that roams in darkness nor the devastating
>   plague at noon.
> You have the Lord for your refuge; you have made the Most
>   High your stronghold. Because you cling to me, I will
>   deliver you; You shall call upon me and I will answer
>   you.
> I will be with you in distress; I will deliver you and glorify
>   you, with length of days I will gratify you and will show
>   you my salvation.

REFERENCES

Arieti, S. *The Intrapsychic Self.* New York: Basic Books, 1967.

Campbell, J. *The Power of Myth with Bill Moyers.* Edited by Betty Sue Flowers. New York: Doubleday, 1988.

Maslow, A.H. Health as Transcendence of Environment. *Journal of Humanistic Psychology* 1:1-5, 1961.

Response to
"The Role of Mental Health
in Spiritual Growth"

I'm neither a theologian nor a psychoanalyst. The dialogue as presented by Dr. Father Smith has been framed in terms of those two disciplines. I will try to broaden that beyond psychoanalysis to the modern world of psychiatry.

I was trained by the Jesuits, and subsequently trained as a psychologist and can identify very much with John Polan's wife (see his remarks). I was always the one who was asking, "How come? How do you know this?" What I like about the Jesuits is that they do that, too. One of my most cherished stories, and it is almost of mythical proportions in my mind, occurred around 1616. The Pope was after Galileo, and in fact told Galileo that he must quit the science stuff and fiddling around with the way the universe is organized. At the very same time, do you know where the Jesuits were? They were in China using modern astronomy to get in favor with the court in China. So there's no doubt that Dr. Father Smith comes from a long line of optimists.

I want to propose a different model from Dr. Smith. I am going to argue for the sake of argument, that there are times when we must keep faith out. There are times when we must bring faith in. I am not sure I agree with this; I am not sure you will, but we can try. Let me give you two instances in which I think it is strategically important for the therapist to keep faith out.

[Haworth co-indexing entry note]: *"Response* to "The Role of Mental Health in Spiritual Growth.""" Clarkin, John F. Co-published simultaneously in the *Journal of Religion in Disability & Rehabilitation* (The Haworth Press, Inc.) Vol. 1, No. 2, 1994, pp. 41-44; and: *Pastoral Care of the Mentally Disabled: Advancing Care of the Whole Person* (ed: Sally K. Severino, and The Reverend Richard Liew) The Haworth Press, Inc., 1994, pp. 41-44. Multiple copies of this article/chapter may be purchased from The Haworth Document Delivery Center [1-800-3-HAWORTH; 9:00 a.m. - 5:00 p.m. (EST)].

41

Some of my work is done with couples in which one partner has bipolar disorder, i.e., manic-depressive illness. Couples who are trying to cope with this genetic, biological, vulnerable situation experience great distress. In one particular case, the husband, a 28-year-old man, was affected and had gone through about five or six serious manic episodes in which he typically would get hypomanic, begin reading the Bible, begin thinking that God was talking to him, and that he was having a religious experience. He would leave home and go to communities across the USA, visiting churches, calling his wife on occasion. He would finally get himself incarcerated so somebody could get lithium into his body.

Our role, it seems to me, is to try to convince this man that we are psychotherapists, "mental illness people" if you will, and that while he may have been having a religious experience, something else was also occurring. In fact, I would argue for a team effort. We called in his minister and his wife and all tried to convince him that, at the very least, he was also influenced by manic-depressive illness. As a result of our efforts, the next time he felt the urge to start visiting churches, we were able to prevent it. All our interventions were in the context, I think, of respect for faith, not interference with faith, but keeping the boundaries clear.

I think Dr. Smith's story is in some ways related to both this first example and the next one I would like to share, concerning a man and woman who were referred to me. The man was an important religious and community leader. We will call him a Protestant minister. In my assessment, and in the assessment of the referring physician, the man was seriously disturbed. He believed his wife was unfaithful to him, was indeed obsessed with this idea. He brought audio tapes to the sessions, tapes he had made secretly as his wife moved around in the kitchen, and he interpreted all of the movements as sexual ones with other partners. This man was very adept at religion, faith and scriptures, and was quite clever at using those in defending his irrational beliefs. It would have come as no surprise if he had demanded that his wife be taken out into the community square, as in Old Testament times, and stoned to death for her adultery. In my assessment of his wife, I found her to be a profound, religious and wonderful person. Her husband needed to be confronted on a human level about serious psychopathology in terms of what he was projecting onto this woman, but religion had to be kept out of the psychotherapy. He was using religion to support his irrationality, disregarding its real meaning and place in life.

When do we bring faith into psychotherapy? I very much feel lifted by Dr. Smith's optimism. Out of contrariness, however, I will introduce some pessimism. I was privileged to hear James Watson lecture last year at the American Psychiatric Association on the Genome Project. The most fascinating thing to come out of that project is the promise that in the near future and from birth we will be able to have a blood test and know what kind of illnesses and diseases are imbedded in our genes. My pessimistic thought is that, despite American democracy, we do not start out as equals. We do not have equal opportunities. In fact, modern psychiatry would suggest that wired into our very biology are differences which do have implications for things like bipolar disorder.

But where do we bring faith in? I think those of us who work with the mentally ill need faith all the time. Without faith, how can we help a 35-year-old, successful man who has manic-depressive illness, and who now feels his career is over, cut short because of his disease? He can no longer concentrate, but must sit and mourn the loss of the person he used to be. What does that mean to him? What kind of meaning can we help him see in that? What does it mean to a mother who has a daughter, a medical student, a very intelligent medical student, who has a psychotic breakdown, the first breakdown in an illness whose prognosis generally can assume there will be others? Who is God and where does God come in? Who allows this situation where it is not all equal?

Dr. Father Smith's model embodies the integration of psychotherapy and spiritual growth. In the beautiful and extraordinary case he described, a young man, who at first was hostile and anxious, in the atmosphere of psychotherapy could begin to look at positive aspects about himself. Psychotherapy is a humble enterprise. It has to do with man's relationship with man. Theology has to do with man's relationship with God. The question, it seems to me, is how do we integrate their efforts? The answer is not faith or mental health; clearly it is faith *and* mental health. But how do we integrate the delivery of services to our patients, who indeed must integrate both?

I am suggesting to you that, while Dr. Father Smith presents one wonderful integrated model, there is a need of a model for a multi-disciplinary staff context wherein the role of spiritual caregiver is clearly differentiated.

John F. Clarkin, PhD

Response to "The Role of Mental Health in Spiritual Growth"

In preparing for today, I played around with the title and I realized how broad the subject is. The role of mental health in spiritual growth: Which, mental health or spiritual growth, is dependant on the other? Does spiritual growth depend on our mental health? If we are having emotional problems, does that interfere with our spiritual growth? Does our mental health depend on our spiritual growth? If we are having spiritual problems, does that mean we are going to have problems with our mental health? I do not really know how to answer those questions, but I have some thoughts about the environments that are helpful to us emotionally as we grow spiritually.

If we read the Gospel of Mark, we eventually understand that Jesus is advising moderation in the religious boundaries we set for ourselves: they need to be neither too rigid nor too unstructured. The kingdom of God is not to be found in slavish adherence to doctrine, but neither is it revealed when we have no firm beliefs or convictions. The man named Job is an example of someone who was fragmented and very loose and needed structure and clear boundaries in his life. On the other hand, Jesus was constantly suggesting that the leaders of his day who were concerned about adherence to the law were too caught up in tight structures and needed to loosen up if they expected to see the kingdom of God.

The parable of the good Samaritan is an example of this. The

[Haworth co-indexing entry note]: *"Response* to "The Role of Mental Health in Spiritual Growth." " Wyrtzen, The Rev. James C. Co-published simultaneously in the *Journal of Religion in Disability & Rehabilitation* (The Haworth Press, Inc.) Vol. 1, No. 2, 1994, pp. 45-48; and: *Pastoral Care of the Mentally Disabled: Advancing Care of the Whole Person* (ed: Sally K. Severino, and The Reverend Richard Liew) The Haworth Press, Inc., 1994, pp. 45-48. Multiple copies of this article/ chapter may be purchased from The Haworth Document Delivery Center [1-800-3-HAWORTH; 9:00 a.m. - 5:00 p.m. (EST)].

45

religious leaders who passed down the road carefully avoided the man who had been beaten by thieves, lest he die and they would be ritually unpure and unable to celebrate the Sabbath. A Samaritan, a rejected half-breed, stopped and cared for the man, leaving money for his recuperation at a local inn. Who among these will see the kingdom of God? My point is, for some people, tight and rigid religious structures are very important for their spiritual growth because they provide an important external structure. Within a rigid external structure they are able to find security and potential for spiritual growth. The same environment may suffocate and stifle other people who need a religious environment which encourages experiencing the creative spirit of God in different ways.

In my work as a pastoral counselor I often see clients search for a spiritual home that provides them an environment of comfort and the potential for growth. Some need an environment that will provide external structure and some need an environment that will encourage freedom and the exploration of creativity. There are many different variations of this along the way. I am in an unusual position as a pastoral counselor, one different from that of pastor. I no longer feel I represent a faith group in which my role is to encourage people's involvement in that group. Instead, I find myself encouraging clients to follow the direction of their instincts, to find the kind of structure that will meet their needs.

At the recent Board of Governors meeting of the American Association of Pastoral Counselors, I was struck by the changes occurring in several of the people in the group. Two of my colleagues were moving from Southern Baptist churches to Episcopal churches in their spiritual struggle to find a home that allowed them to express themselves. One was moving from a Brethren church, a rigid structure, to an American Baptist church, a more flexible structure. Another colleague was leaving the United Church of Christ to become a Roman Catholic because he felt he needed that kind of shift in order to express himself. Each change represents the need for an environment in which the spirit can grow comfortably and within a structure that allows each person to seek the kingdom of God in peace.

The second point I want to make is that, the way we think about life and the way we view life makes the real difference. If we see life as a spiritual journey and a spiritual experience, life will be very much defined by this and different because of this. The values we carry within ourselves about life and about people very much define the way we approach life and the way we approach the persons to whom we minister. I think of pastoral counseling as a spiritual journey and a spiritual experience. I believe understanding what we are experiencing, feeling and struggling with is one of the deepest spiritual experiences in life. Whether I am talking about something that sounds religious or not, that religious, spiritual value is present.

As pastoral counselors we are in an interaction in which we, the client and the creative spirit of God are all present and actively creating something greater than what is going on in the room. We are creating an environment where a change in growth can take place. To me, pastoral counseling is a way of helping to improve mental health, but in the context of a spiritual health that can also be made better. I was struck by the definition of "optimism" and "pro-actively." I pulled back within myself and said, "For some reason that doesn't feel right to me, yet that's always the way I perceived myself–very optimistic and very proactive." But then I heard the words about having essential needs met. I thought about that. So many people with whom I sit every day of the week have not had their essential needs met. As a result, they are coming to counseling with very deep conflicts and struggles. My role is to understand and be present and to find some kind of optimism or pro-activity within the process.

My associations go back 25 years, to my last year of seminary and an inter-seminary seminar project. It included seven different seminaries and each chose two people to meet for a semester and a half every Friday afternoon. The seminar I was assigned to was on atheism. Everyone was eager to read Hegel, or Althizer or Descarte in order to write a paper about atheism. I had been a philosophy minor in college and had come to the conclusion that my representational systems and philosophy were definitely not similar. I was sitting there thinking, "Oh God . . . do I have to go back and do Hegel again?", when the question was asked, "Would anybody like to do a biblical study on atheism?" I volunteered.

The seminary I attended emphasized biblical languages and I had majored in Hebrew, Aramaic and Greek. I began with the Hebrew scriptures and did a Hebrew word study of all the words related to faith and lack of faith. Then I went to the New Testament and did a Greek word study of all the words that related to faith and lack of faith. As a result of the study, I realized, in the Greek word study all the first generation literature has " 'o pistos"–"faith" or "the faith." But in the second generation literature, the word is "pisteo-men"–"we believe." What was faith to the first generation was translated as beliefs in the second generation.

This says something about the relationship between mental and spiritual belief and faith. When I go into the therapy room and work with my clients, sometimes I get confused about what I believe. After ten years of graduate school and two decades of experience as a counselor, I find I often am not sure what to do. The struggle is in finding the right intervention and enabling the client to look within himself/herself to find that place for growth and health. But what remains true and constant is my faith in the person with whom I am working. That is where the optimism is.

The Reverend James C. Wyrtzen, DMin

Anton Boisen:
Madness, Mental Health and the Ministry

The Reverend Curtis W. Hart MDiv

INTRODUCTION:
BACKGROUND AND SHAPING FORCES

Erik Erikson uses a quote attributed to the young Martin Luther: "I did not learn my theology all at once but I had to search deeper for it where my temptations took me" (Erikson, 1958, p. 251). Erikson then continues with his own commentary on these words of the 16th-century Reformer: "A theologian is born by living, nay dying and being damned not by thinking, reading or speculating" (Erikson, 1958, p. 251).

While Erikson here alludes to young Luther's inner conflicts and his protracted identity crisis, his description could also be applied to Anton Theophilus Boisen (October 29, 1876-October 1, 1965). Both individuals shared a disposition for rumination and scholarship and were possessed by deep inner struggles. Both lived, acted and wrote in eras of important cultural and religious transition. And both occupied a central role in founding movements where their contributions continue to be revered and debated.

Anton Boisen was a child of Victorian America and its 19th-century Protestant culture. He was a deeply disturbed human being "whose autobiography contains descriptions of six psychotic episodes during the thirty-seven years from 1898 to 1935." (Thornton,

[Haworth co-indexing entry note]: "Anton Boisen: Madness, Mental Health and the Ministry." Hart, The Reverend Curtis W. Co-published simultaneously in the *Journal of Religion in Disability & Rehabilitation* (The Haworth Press, Inc.) Vol. 1, No. 2, 1994, pp. 49-65; and: *Pastoral Care of the Mentally Disabled: Advancing Care of the Whole Person* (ed: Sally K. Severino, and The Reverend Richard Liew) The Haworth Press, Inc., 1994, pp. 49-65. Multiple copies of this article/chapter may be purchased from The Haworth Document Delivery Center [1-800-3-HAWORTH; 9:00 a.m. - 5:00 p.m. (EST)].

49

1970, p. 55). The first mental hospital chaplain in America, he was a prolific writer who produced three major books in his lifetime as well as numerous articles. He inspired and edited a hymnal and service book for use in hospitals and was the founding figure in the movement providing clinical training to clergy in health care settings (known officially since 1967 as Clinical Pastoral Education).

Central to an understanding of Boisen's life and work lies the realization stemming from his own encounter with mental illness. Reflecting on that experience in 1950, he wrote: "I believe that certain forms of mental illness, particularly those characterized by anxiety and conviction of sin, are not evils. They are instead manifestations of the power that makes for health. They are analogous to fever or inflammation in the body. I am thus very sure that the experience which plunged me into this new field of labor was mental illness of the most profound and unmistakable variety. I am equally sure that it was for me a problem-solving religious experience. My efforts to follow the leads derived from my own experience and checking them against the experience of others has convinced me that my experience was by no means unique. . . . I believe that the real evil in functional mental illness is not to be found in discontent with one's imperfections, even when that discontent is carried to the point of severe disturbance, but in the sense of estrangement and isolation due to the presence of instinctual claims which can neither be controlled nor acknowledged for fear of condemnation. The aim of psychotherapy is not to get rid of the conflict by lowering the conscience threshold but to remove the sense of alienation by restoring the sufferer to the internalized fellowship of the best and thus setting him free to strive for his true objectives in life" (Boisen, 1960, pp. 196-197).

Beginning in 1925 Boisen taught pastoral care and counseling to theological students and clergy, first at Worcester (Massachusetts) State Hospital and after 1932 at Elgin (Illinois) State Hospital. He sought to help his students develop a sympathetic understanding of what it was like to live in what he called "the wilderness of the lost."

In these endeavors Boisen became convinced, even obsessed, by what this clinical experience might mean for the church and its ministers. He put it this way in 1951: "Let me also emphasize the fact that our movement, as I have conceived of it, has no new gospel to proclaim. We are not even seeking to introduce anything new into the theological curriculum beyond a new approach to some ancient programs. We are trying, rather, to call attention back to the central task of the church, that of 'saving souls,' and to the central problem of theology, that of sin and salvation. What is new is the attempt to begin with the study of living human documents rather than with books and to focus attention upon those who are grappling desperately with the issues of spiritual life and death" (Thornton, 1970, p. 64).

These two beliefs, first, that mental illness has a profoundly spiritual and potentially creative character and, second, that encounters with the "living human documents" of those suffering dysfunction and disorder was a necessary cornerstone of theological education, propelled Boisen's professional life from 1922 onward.

It is critical to note that these core insights came when Anton Boisen was well into middle life. His career as a mental hospital chaplain began in 1925 when he was forty-eight years old. His major writings (his three major books, the hymnal he edited, and seventy-one of his seventy-nine articles) appear after this date.

Of the three books, his first, *The Exploration of the Inner World: A Study of Mental Disorder and Religious Experience,* took up the relation between religion and mental health from Boisen's unique perspective as minister, theologian, chaplain and patient. He introduced his themes with words reflecting his belief that: "This I shall do with the ever deepening conviction that only as we study the one in the light of the other shall we be able to understand either one or to gain any insight into the laws of the spiritual life with which theology and psychiatry are equally concerned" (Boisen, 1936, p. 11).

In this book he utilized a case method approach then new to the theological enterprise. Among the cases he considered was that of George Fox, founder of the Society of Friends, whom Boisen believed experienced the isolation of mental disorder. Boisen saw this experience as a necessary and creative step in Fox's becoming the leader of a new religious group infused with the fresh perspective of what Quakers call the "inner light." Boisen saw Fox as a "living human document" worthy of study. Fox was also a figure with whom Boisen closely identified. Boisen's empirical approach to religious experience drew upon and made use of his own struggles (e.g., his chapter on the Messianic consciousness of religious leaders) in an effort to understand others. *The Exploration of the Inner World* was as much an opportunity to demonstrate Boisen's emerging clinical theology as it was an occasion to discuss his view of psychiatric disturbance as potentially purposeful.

Boisen's second major book, *Religion in Crisis and Custom,* was in many ways the synthesis of material arising from essays and articles written in the period 1925-1955, and showed how convinced Boisen was of the relevance of science and the scientific method in the study of religious movements, figures and trends. This focus upon sciences and religion began for Boisen in his work with George Albert Coe, Professor of Religious Education, while he was a student at Union Theological Seminary. Even in that era of American theological education (1908-1911), Coe saw the need for a dynamic psychology of religion that had practical applications.

The content of both these books suggested how much Boisen was shaped in his formative years and productive adult period by the spirit of liberal Protestantism. Though not an official school of thought, the impact of liberalism was felt throughout the Protestant churches in latter nineteenth- and early twentieth-century America. Theological liberalism was the reigning intellectual force of Boisen's "creative milieu." Two major historians of the pastoral care movement place him within the orbit of its influence. According to one of them (Allison Stokes), "liberalism's central characteristics are (1) cultural accommodations, (2) God's immanence and (3) pro-gressivism" (Stokes, 1985, pp. 149-159). These characteristics stress the indivisibility of the sacred and the secular, the need for a pluralistic outlook in the search for ultimate truth, a belief in the primacy of the human experience of God as a basis for any theology and an implicit faith in modern modes of scientific inquiry as a basis for the improvement of the world and the pursuit of truth. Clearly, the spirit of this liberal world view made possible not only the reception of Boisen's clinical approach to theology but also provided the backdrop for the ensuing dialogue between psychiatry and religion. Its spirit, moveover, made certain that the liberal Protestant world could receive the work of Freud and his followers as it crossed the Atlantic and found its way into academic and popular circles.

The last of Boisen's books is his autobiography, *Out of the Depths,* published in 1960 when he was turning eighty-four. The title was a reference to Psalm 130 ("Out of the depths I have called to Thee, O Lord; Lord hear my cry . . . my soul waits for the Lord more eagerly than watchmen for the morning" [vss. 1,6, NEB]). This volume described in detail Boisen's sensitive nature and episodes of illness. It was his most extensive case history, the place where his clinical theology found its most detailed exposition. As such, it was at turns as sad, courageous, revealing and opaque as the solitary man who produced it.

EARLY LIFE: LOSSES AND NEW DIRECTIONS (1876-1920)

Boisen's autobiography revealed a family life shaped by Victorian morality and Protestant religiosity. Both his parents were regular attenders of the Presbyterian church into which their firstborn and only son would later be ordained. Teaching and the ministry were the vocations pursued on both sides of the family for three generations prior to Anton's birth in October of 1876. His earliest years were spent in Bloomington, Indiana where his father taught modern languages and botany at Indiana University. Hermann Boisen was a German immigrant who came to the United States in 1869 to pursue an academic career. He was described by his son this way: "My father was the dominant member of the household. He was always full of life and full of ideas, interested in everything that went on. His was a contagious enthusiasm which carried others along with him. He was a great lover of nature, of trees and shrubs and flowers, and he took great interest in teaching me the names of the trees. . . . He could be stern but he was always kind. On two occasions which I can recall, the offense was lying. I do not remember what it was about, but I do remember his explaining very carefully why I was being punished and how many blows I was to receive. He always set a maximum and a minimum, the minimum being employed if I refrained from crying. He was always careful to make it clear that there was no change in his love for me and that the punishment was not arbitrary but a necessary consequence of what I had done" (Boisen, 1960, p. 23). This experience of paternal love was to have great impact on Anton's adult beliefs and relationships.

His mother, Louise Wylie Boisen, was described as being gifted in music and devoted to the care of her home and children. Her manner is recounted as: " . . . gentle and forbearing. Throughout her dealing with me she relied on persuasion rather than compulsion. She made me feel bad when I did not do as I ought to do" (Boisen, 1960, p. 23).

Louise Boisen was one of the first women admitted to the University of Indiana, from which she graduated in 1871. After a stint as a college teacher, she returned to Bloomington to marry Hermann who had been her instructor there. Boisen viewed his mother as a model of piety, self-giving love, high ideals and self-control. These were qualities he endeavored to emulate and later found embodied in the woman with whom he would maintain a sustained relationship.

Boisen's sister, Marie, was born in 1879 when Anton was two years and eleven months old. His writing shows how envious he was of his sister, though this envy was expressed in a muted tone. In high school he was shy and reclusive, scared of talking about sex even with his friends. Marie, on the other hand, was warm, outgoing, the most popular girl in her class. She was, it seems, everything her brother was not.

Boisen's father was an itinerant academic. Having no Ph.D., he moved from appointment to appointment. It was during the time that Hermann Boisen was teaching at the Lawrenceville School in New Jersey that he suffered a heart attack and died in 1883 at the age of 38. Anton was then seven years old. The grief elicited by his father's death was intense. Boisen wrote: "His memory, influenced by my mother's picture of him and that of others who knew him, has remained a potent force in my life, one which for me has been associated with my idea of God" (Boisen, 1960, p. 27).

It is worth noting that the God addressed in the prayers written and collected for the hymnal and service book (first called *Lift Up Your Hearts,* later entitled *Hymns of Hope and Courage*) Boisen edited in the 1920's reveals qualities similar to those of Hermann Boisen: demanding and loving, deserving of praise, full of forgiveness but expecting always finer things from His followers. One suspects that memories of Hermann Boisen were kept alive and reinforced by Louise's recollections and that they gradually became enshrined in the family history.

The Boisens returned to Bloomington from New Jersey following Hermann's sudden death. There Anton attended local public schools and the Presbyterian Church. Never in the autobiography is there a suggestion of any major rebellion from the standards and values of school, church or extended family. Whatever criticism he might have held in the area of religious belief would have to wait until age 32, when he entered into full-time study for the ministry.

Anton Boisen attended the University of Indiana and studied romance languages (his mother's field), which he taught there upon graduation. This interest faded and he turned elsewhere. For some years his love of nature compelled an interest in forestry. To fulfill that interest he attended the Yale School of Forestry for a year but did not complete the degree. Forestry, along with pursuit of an academic position, became the second career he abandoned.

During the year 1905, while living in New Haven, Anton made his decision to enter the ministry. His call was the culmination of considerable reflection over many years, coupled with intense moments of encounter with words of Scripture. This era of inner reflection for him dated from Easter 1898. Three of these periods of intense reflection were marked by experiences whose descriptions suggest temporary psychotic states. Boisen's recounting of them included feelings of having become engulfed, overwhelmed and detached from reality. They were filled with what Boisen perceived to be signs of a mystical sort.

Whatever their character, Boisen emerged aware, intact and coherent enough to pursue his call to the ministry to the doors of Union Theological Seminary in New York, which he entered in 1908. Always in need of approval, he remembers: "To this change of cause [from forestry] my mother gave her full consent and helped make it possible" (Boisen, 1960, p. 58).

Boisen wrote of his decision to enter the ministry to Alice Batchelder whom he had met on the Indiana campus in 1902. He described his first encounter with her in this extended passage: "She was an Easterner, a native of Portsmouth, New Hampshire, and a graduate of Smith College, who came to Indiana University in 1902 as Secretary of the Young Women's Christian Association. I saw her for the first time at a convocation, where she was introduced to the student body and made a brief address. She was at the time twenty-two years of age. She was somewhat above average height, with wavy hair of genuine golden color. What she said I do not remember, but she spoke in a clear, well-modulated voice, and I was impressed with her sincerity and earnestness. I fell in love with her then and there. It was a one-sided affair, a love that swept me off my feet. I received little encouragement, but I saw her from time to time as often as she would let me" (Boisen, 1960, p. 52).

Anton pursued Alice for years. She was the embodiment of a dream of fulfillment for him: physical beauty, intellect, pristine values, the potential ideal life partner of a successful, secure parish pastor. This dream of Anton's was not to find in Alice a willing, earthly accomplice. She rebuffed his advances and declarations of love. For some time she refused to see him or respond to the letters he would send to her on a daily basis.

Alice Batchelder never married and sustained an ambivalent relationship with Anton Boisen until her death from cancer in 1935. The pursuit of her love was for him a powerful force. Retrospectively, he saw his call to the ministry as being connected to his desire to win Alice over by proving his virtue and demonstrating his need for her. Her idealized image dominated his thoughts. Though this relationship was most probably never consummated, the sense of wonder she elicited in Anton maintained an elusive and powerful authority over his life. The relationship between Anton and Alice may be seen as similar to that of Kierkegaard and Regina Olsen. As the theologian Henri Nouwen provocatively asks, in this case, "Are we dealing with an adolescent love affair or a therapeutic relationship?" (Nouwen, 1968, p. 56).

Boisen's abiding love for Alice was expressed in the dedication of his first book, *The Exploration of the Inner World,* published a year after Alice's death: "TO THE MEMORY OF A.L.B. For her sake I undertook the adventure out of which this book has grown. Her compassion upon a wretch in direst need, her wisdom and courage and unanswering fidelity have made possible the measure of success which may have been achieved. To her I dedicate it in the name of the Love which would surmount every barrier, and bridge every chasm and make sure the foundations of the universe" (Boisen, 1936, Dedication).

It would be easy to dismiss these words as a painful expression of grief and unrequited love. The fact is, however, that Anton Boisen took Alice–or more correctly, his idealized image of her –with him into the depths and out. She was thus to be his companion on the lonely journey that reached its central crisis in 1920 when Boisen was first hospitalized and after which his period of greatest influence and activity began.

AN EXPLORER
IN A "LITTLE KNOWN COUNTRY" (1920-1935)

Anton Boisen's life journey led him three times to be hospitalized for mental illness. The first occasion was in 1920; writing a statement of belief required of candidates seeking ministerial positions, he found himself absorbed and later so distraught that family members moved to have him committed. The experience of living in a "little known country," as he called it, was fully, even exhaustively described in *Out of The Depths*. Like the first hospitalization in 1920, the other two in 1930 and 1935 were followed by periods of intense intellectual and professional activity. These latter hospitalizations took place after the death of Boisen's mother, Louise, in 1930 and after the death of Alice Batchelder in 1935. Edward Thornton reports that "Boisen remained symptom free from age fifty-nine until his death at eighty-eight on October 1, 1965" (Thornton, 1970, p. 58). During this span he was looked after and cared for by former students and staff at Elgin (Illinois) State Hospital, where he came to work in 1932. He lived out his last years in semiretirement in a small suite of rooms at Elgin, a short distance from the wards where he had worked as a chaplain and similar to the ones where he had been hospitalized and treated.

Before his first hospitalization, Boisen had an undistinguished nine-year career in the ministry after graduating from Union Seminary in 1911. He engaged in sociological research into the life of rural churches, was the pastor of small churches himself, and for a short while served as a campus minister in Ames, Iowa. It was clear that, though intellectually gifted, for the third time he was unsuccessful in choosing a career.

On October 9, 1920, his life abruptly changed. While visiting his sister, Marie, in Arlington, Massachusetts, Boisen became remote and was clearly disturbed. Admitted first to Boston Psychopathic Hospital and transferred one week later to Westboro State Hospital, he fell into a state of profound disorganization. He experienced wild, racing thoughts, an agitated mood and a collection of strange perceptions of the world that were not under his control. The record of his stay is harrowing and poignant. Boisen recorded it first for a graduate course he took two and a half years after discharge from the hospital and it appeared again in *Out of The Depths*. Within this extended passage are Boisen's memories of staff, patients and the special meanings he attached to random occurrences. Included are examples of religious symbolism and ideas that erupted and caught his attention. Among them are the Day of Judgement, the search for the Holy Grail and Boisen's attempt to rearrange the world according to the pattern of a cosmic harmony he called the Family of Four.

Friends were frightened for him. They wrote him and he responded. They tried to have him moved at one point of relative calm to Bloomingdale Hospital in White Plains, New York where he was to receive analytic treatment. Suffering a relapse, Boisen was not able to leave Westboro and was, in fact, returned to a locked ward where his most acute symptoms reappeared. This hospitalization lasted until January of 1922. When finally discharged, Boisen went to stay with his friend, Norman Nash, then teaching at the Episcopal Theological School in Cambridge, Massachusetts.

Boisen's diagnosis at Westboro was, by his description, schizophrenic reaction, catatonic type.

Psychiatrist and historian Robert C. Powell sheds light on Boisen's diagnosis with this extended comment:

> The question of Boisen's diagnosis is not academic, for the theory of schizophrenia he later proposed, though supported by the observations of psychiatrist Harry Stack Sullivan, first came to Boisen through an analysis of his own case. In brief, Boisen suggested that certain forms of psychosis represent problem solving attempts at cure and reorganization, which are closely related to certain forms of profound religious expe-

rience. Since Boisen's theory rested on a sharp differentiation of catatonia from other subgroups of schiziophrenia the crucial question is, 'Was Boisen's a case of catatonia?'

Assuming for a moment that Boisen's behavior was catatonic, it is unfortunate for the inquiring layman that *Webster's New Collegiate Dictionary* defines "catatonia" as "a disorder marked by catalepsy," and then defines "catalepsy" as "a condition of suspended animation and loss of voluntary motion in which the limbs hold any position they are placed in." Webster's definition holds true for only half of the broader syndrome, which includes both "stuporous catatonia," described by Webster's, and "excited catatonia," which may have characterized Boisen's disturbance. As Hinsie and Campbell's *Psychiatric Dictionary* notes, "The clinical syndrome called catatonia is characterized as a rule by (1) stupor, associated with either marked rigidity or flexibility of the musculature or (2) overactivity in conjunction with various manifestations of stereotype. . . . It is true that catatonia or rather cataleptoid syndromes are not infrequently a part of other diagnostic groups (e.g., hysteria and manic-depressive psychosis), but the tendency is to restrict the term catatonia to the schizophrenic group." This last clause should be emphasized, for the descriptions of Boisen's behavior do prompt one to consider "manic-depressive psychosis, manic phase" as a possible diagnosis.

In any case, Dr. Milton H. Erickson, Boisen's psychiatrist in 1930 and confidante in later years, has emphasized Boisen's problem as a disorder of thought rather than of affect, and as catatonic rather than paranoid. Psychoanalytic psychologists David Shakow and Paul Pruyser both feel confident of Erickson's diagnosis. Shakow had intermittent contact with Boisen—as a fellow student, colleague and friend–from 1923 on, while Pruyser knew Boisen after 1958 and has already commented in print on the increasingly flat nature of Boisen's affect.

Thus, although there undoubtedly were excessively affective components to Boisen's behavior during his disturbed episodes, one may feel some confidence in his self-diagnosis of 'dementia praecox, catatonia.' (Powell, 1974, p. 133)

Though it might be that a diagnosis of affective disorder is suggested by the evidence, we can safely maintain that the designation of a cognitive disorder is justified given the testimony of clinicians who knew Boisen personally.

Whatever label his behavior, mood and thinking warrant, Boisen felt that at Westboro he had passed through a period of transformation in which he had, as he wrote, "broken an opening in the wall that separated medicine and religion" (Boisen, 1960, p. 91). Once returned to relatively sound health, Boisen was energized, even compelled, to learn all he could about dynamic psychiatry and to share his experience with all who would listen.

Though Boisen believed his psychiatric illness to have religious meaning, he was at the same time aware of its dynamic components, namely the failure of his relationship with Alice and his struggle with his own sexuality. While he noted these causative dynamic forces, there is little detailed evidence of how, when and why Boisen came to these conclusions. He also showed awareness of the severity of his own conscience (superego). Because the demands of his conscience were so severe, Boisen was never able to find relaxation or fulfillment in intimacy and sexual gratification.

Boisen returned temporarily to academic life (Harvard, Episcopal Theological School) to reconstruct the learning from his recent past. His motivation was understandable, given the location of his recovery in the Nash home and the fact that it was in an academic environment that he had met more success and felt greater security than any other place in his life. He decided a return to the parish ministry was not possible after what he had been through. He needed a new avenue to find fulfillment, self-expression and self-esteem.

Three physicians, along with friends and students, became central to Boisen's emerging enterprise. The first, Richard Clarke Cabot, M.D., of the Massachusetts General Hospital and the Harvard Medical School, met Boisen while he was attending seminars in his post-hospitalization period. Cabot had been a pioneer in the clinical case method in the teaching of physicians and he became fascinated with Boisen's interest in helping the sick. Perhaps the clinical case method might have some relevance for clergy. Cabot later became disillusioned with Boisen's preoccupations regarding the psychogenesis of mental illness and its spiritual or religious meaning, and was deeply upset by Boisen's psychotic episode of 1930. He nonetheless was instrumental in making it possible for Boisen to pursue his interests by introducing him and recommending him as a chaplain to William Byran, M.D., who was the superintendent of Worcester (Massachusetts) State Hospital.

Cabot first encouraged Boisen to learn about and utilize the case method himself. Some of the fruits of those labors are evident in *The Exploration of the Inner World*. Moreover, the method was incorporated into the teaching of seminarians whom Boisen later recruited and brought to Worcester. The clinical training of ministers and theological students is much indebted to this patrician New Englander. Cabot published "Plea for a Clinical Year in the course of Theological Study" (1925) and in 1930 it was at Cabot's Brattle Street home that the charter of the Council for Clinical Training for Theological Students was signed and incorporated. The first chaplain at Massachusetts General Hospital, Russell Dicks, once noted, "the Cabots were reputed to have a private line of communication with God. I always suspected Richard Cabot really believed that" (Thornton, 1970, p. 46).

Cabot did not agree with Boisen's psychological and religious ideas regarding mental illness. Perhaps that was because he was convinced of their biological causation. It may be, however, as Allison Stokes has noted, "that his discomfort with Boisen's ideas stemmed from the fact that he (Cabot) had a sibling who was a chronic manic-depressive and he had tired or remained thoroughly unconvinced of psychological explanations of this and other psychiatric conditions" (Stokes, 1985, p. 49).

It was William A. Byran, M.D., who accepted Boisen as a chaplain at Worcester in 1924. In so doing, he showed the same independence of mind and willingness to risk that Cabot had shown in embarking on this new activity with Boisen only three years after a major hospitalization. Byran was among a handful of leaders in American psychiatry who early on supported and actively cultivated the clinical training movement. Other psychiatrist administrators who were to occupy a similar role in the clinical training of clergy were Arthur P. Noyes, M.D., of Norristown (Pennsylvania) State Hospital, Winifred Overholser, M.D., of St. Elizabeth's Hospital, Washington, D.C., and Karl Menninger, M.D., of the Menninger Clinic, Topeka, Kansas.

Students came to Worcester for the summer. They were ward attendants during the day shift, and their evenings were spent discussing cases with Boisen. They planned activities and led programs for patients, including worship services. In meetings with the clinical staff they talked about their experiences; they also participated in research projects. Most of the students were white, male and represented the Eastern and progressive (liberal) seminaries: Union, Yale, Harvard, Boston University, Episcopal Theological School. One exception was Helen Flanders Dunbar, then a student at Union. Her relationship with Boisen evolved from mentorship into friendship and later, collaboration. Flanders Dunbar (she dropped her first name professionally) is described as an "intellectual Amazon" (Thornton, 1970, p. 77) because along with the two degree programs already mentioned, she went on to pursue medical training at Yale and psychiatric residency before gaining prominence in the area of psychosomatics.

Some have speculated that there was more than intellectual and professional fraternity in the relationship between Dunbar and Boisen. While any romantic attachment seems improbable, given Boisen's commitment to Alice Batchelder, Dunbar retained a powerful role in Boisen's life and in that of the clinical training movement. She became the first Medical Director of the Council for Clinical Training for Theological Students in 1930 and was also instrumental in encouraging the dialogue between religion and medicine as the head of a joint committee of the Federal Council of Churches and the New York Academy of Medicine that "helped promote psychosomatic understanding in the United States" (Stokes, 1985, p. 77).

For Boisen's part, he obviously delighted in having a student so gifted, one knowledgeable in theological matters and about to go into medicine and psychiatry. Moreover, Dunbar's Ph.D. dissertation concerned Dante, who was for Boisen something of a patron saint. She also shared his interest in the research that was then emerging in his writings.

It may be that Flanders Dunbar assumed some of the caretaking functions Boisen always hoped would be Alice's lot. She was in many ways his muse and his helpmate. Thus, Dunbar may have become psychologically merged with Alice in a way that encouraged him to go on about the business of teaching, writing and convincing others of the validity of his religious and educational ideas.

Boisen went to Elgin State Hospital two years after his second hospitalization, in 1930. Both this hospitalization and the one in 1935 were of relatively short duration (in each case, several weeks). He went through a similar pattern of renewed energy and purpose following the cessation of symptoms on both occasions.

At Elgin he taught, wrote and did research at the Chicago Theological Seminary under the watchful eye of the seminary president, Arthur Cushman McGiffert, known to Boisen since his days at Union. Though he was always acknowledged as a "father" to the clinical training movement he was not much of an organizational leader. Those tasks were left to others in the years that followed (1935-1965). Boisen lamented never achieving a satisfactory marital relationship. Because of that failure, he was denied the security of having a family of his own. He found compensation in his latter years in the students and colleagues who helped take care of him. He was able to offer them and others support and counsel. His paternal disposition and kindly nature thus won for him the nickname, "Pappy." While the latter era of Boisen's life was productive, he would spend much of his time after 1936 (the date of publication of *The Exploration of The Inner World*) elaborating and expanding upon the insights, themes and ideas of the previous years.

BOISEN'S LEGACY: CLINICAL THEOLOGIAN AND RELIGIOUS ACTUALIST

Anton Boisen's legacy lies, above all else, in its inspiration of an innovative method in the training of clergy and a spirit of inquiry in the dialogue between religion and psychiatry. While the clinical method Boisen first used with his students at Worcester has undergone considerable modification in theory and practice, its essence remains consistent with the vision of its founder. He warned again and again that without an encounter with persons in crisis ("the living document"), theological ideas, religious rituals and traditional words are empty and trivial. Words like "grace," "repentance," and "forgiveness" become real only in dialogue with human experience. Without such encounters, they become understood as symbols or ideas devoid of meaning and transforming power because they no longer connect human experience to what Paul Tillich calls the Ground of Being Itself.

Boisen demonstrated first in his own life, then shared with the students who became his followers, and finally exposed the larger theological community to the power of his vision and experience. He thus became what Erik Erikson calls a "religious actualist": "The religious actualist . . . inevitably becomes an innovator for his very passion and power will want to make actual for others what actualizes him" (Erikson, 1969, p. 399).

For Boisen, it was his conviction of the importance of encounters with "living human documents" that formed him as an innovator and actualizer in the teaching of theological students. Boisen stressed continually the transforming power of his illness as the key to his productive life and his point of entry into what he metaphorically called "the fellowship of the best." This process of transformation may be likened to what Henri F. Ellenberger calls "creative illness," a process Ellenberger views as operative in the lives of both Freud and Jung. It is outlined as follows:

> This compels us to define creative illness and give its main features. It occurs in various settings and is to be found among shamans, among the mystics of various religions, in certain philosophers and creative writers . . . A creative illness succeeds a period of intense preoccupation with an idea and search for a certain truth. It is a polymorphous condition that can take the shape of depression, neurosis, psychosomatic ailments, or even psychosis. Whatever the symptoms, they are felt as painful, if not agonizing, by the subject, with alternating periods of alleviation and worsening. Throughout the illness the subject never loses the thread of his dominating preoccupation. It is often compatible with normal, professional activity and family life. But even if he keeps to his social activities, he is almost entirely absorbed with himself. He suffers from feelings of utter isolation, even when he has a mentor

who guides him through the ordeal (like the shaman apprentice with his master). The termination is often rapid and marked by a phase of exhilaration. The subject emerges from his ordeal with a permanent transformation in his personality and the conviction that he has discovered a great truth or a new spiritual world. (Ellenberger, 1970, pp. 447-448)

It is not hard to trace this paradigm in Boisen's life and work. His "creative illness" gave to the churches and to American theological education a new direction, a new vocabulary, a new method, a new set of priorities. In this way, Anton Boisen's madness promoted health in American religion and theological education and continues to shape the ministry.

REFERENCES

Boisen, A.T. *The Exploration of the Inner World: A Study of Mental Illness and Religious Experience.* New York: Harper, 1936.
Boisen, A.T. *Religion in Crisis and Custom: A Sociological and Psychological Study.* New York: Harper, 1955.
Boisen, A.T. *Out of The Depths.* New York: Harper, 1960.
Boisen, A.T. (ed.) *Hymns of Hope and Courage.* New York: A. S. Barnes and Company, 1937.
Ellenberger, H.F. *The Discovery of The Unconscious.* New York: Basic Books, 1970.
Erikson, E.H. *Young Man Luther: A Study of Psychoanalysis and History.* New York: Norton, 1958.
Erikson, E.H. *Gandhi's Truth.* New York: Norton, 1969.
LeFevre, P. (ed.) Anton T. Boisen memorial issue. *Pastoral Psychology,* 1968.
Nouwen, H.J.M. Anton T. Boisen and theology through living human documents. *Pastoral Psychology* 19:49-64, 1968.
Powell, R.C. *Healing and Wholeness: Helen Flanders Dunbar (1902-59): An Extra-Medical Origin of the American Psychosomatic Movement, 1906-1936;* unpublished doctoral dissertation, Duke University, pp. 120-151, 1974.
Powell, R.C. *CPE: Fifty Years of Learning Through Supervised Encounter with Human Documents.* New York: Association for Clinical Pastoral Education, Inc., 1975.
Stokes, A. *Ministry After Freud.* New York: Pilgrim Press, 1985.
Thornton, E.E. *Professional Education for Ministry: A History of Clinical Pastoral Education.* New York: Abingdon, 1970.
Wallace, E.R. IV. Psychiatry and Religion: Toward a Dialogue and Public Philosophy in Psychiatry and Humanities: *Psychoanalysis and Religion,* Volume 11. Edited by Smith, J.H., Handelman, S.A. Baltimore: Johns Hopkins University Press, pp. 195-21 X, 1990.

Rage at God and Its Transformation: An Adolescent Male and the Death of His Father from AIDS– An Object Relations Perspective

Vernon J. Gregson, Jr., PhD

As the previous papers and discussions have indicated, our patients do not neatly divide themselves or their issues into our rather clearly delineated specialties. They see themselves as a whole, and it is precisely our recognition of this that has led us to this symposium and to seek the interconnections between our disciplines. Both in ourselves and in our patients we see the live, interconnected issues we are trying to confront theoretically by discussing the relationships of psychology, psychoanalysis, psychiatry and religion.

The original impulse for the type of interdisciplinary approach between psychoanalysis and religion that I practice was in large part stimulated by my training in the Roman Catholic School of Spirituality of Ignatius Loyola and by the research of Ana-Maria Rizzuto, M.D., which is presented in her book, *The Birth of the Living God* (1979). Dr. Rizzuto is a psychiatrist and psychoanalyst who did a study of the image of God in the patients and staff of a psychiatric hospital. Her aim was to discover if Freud's theory was correct–that a person's image of God was really that of his or her protective yet

[Haworth co-indexing entry note]: "Rage at God and Its Transformation: An Adolescent Male and the Death of His Father from AIDS–An Object Relations Perspective." Gregson, Vernon J., Jr. Co-published simultaneously in the *Journal of Religion in Disability & Rehabilitation* (The Haworth Press, Inc.) Vol. 1, No. 2, 1994, pp. 67-77; and: *Pastoral Care of the Mentally Disabled: Advancing Care of the Whole Person* (ed: Sally K. Severino, and The Reverend Richard Liew) The Haworth Press, Inc., 1994, pp. 67-77. Multiple copies of this article/chapter may be purchased from The Haworth Document Delivery Center [1-800-3-HAWORTH; 9:00 a.m. - 5:00 p.m. (EST)].

forbidding father, writ large on the heavens. In her research she precinded from Freud's specific hypothesis about the father and explored more generally the relationship, if any, between people's images of God and their early family contexts. As an aid in her research, and with the recognition that spontaneous drawings can reveal deep levels of the unconscious, she asked people to draw their images of God as well as their images of their family and to discuss their thoughts and feelings about the images. She found remarkable correlations between the two images, which she found to have significant theoretical and diagnostic value. She discovered there were indeed relationships between people's images of God and of their parents; but these relationships were not limited to the image of their fathers, as Freud thought. They also significantly, and often more significantly, involved the mother. And the correlations could involve any, particularly early, developmental stage or issues, not just family romance that Freud called the Oedipal complex. Freud's conjecture, therefore, that our image of God was that of the father had been only partially correct. It did apply to some people's image of God, but by no means to all people.

In my own research and clinical practice, I also seek the relationship between the person's image of God and their early developmental experiences. Unlike Dr. Rizzuto, I ask people to draw their relationship to God rather than their image of God, since I have found that less threatening to many people, for religious or other reasons. I also find I get the same or more information this way. It is the character of the relationship that I am after anyway. Many, however, do draw their images of God as part of expressing their relationship to God.

I also ask Christian clients to draw their relationship to Jesus and their relationship to the Spirit. If they are Roman Catholic, I also ask them to draw their relationship to Mary. There are different constellations of feelings about each of these religious relationships. A person might feel close to God but alienated from Jesus, or vice versa. Different familial relationships can be used for each. Although Dr. Rizzuto worked largely with Christians, I do not think she realized that different issues are addressed in a Christian's relationship to each of the persons of the Christian Trinity. One can miss some important information with only one drawing. Different elements of people's early life experiences are presented in their drawings of these religious relationships, indicating they were formed at different emotionally significant periods and with regard to different persons.

Also unlike Dr. Rizzuto, I have my patients draw both their present families and their families of origin, to see how developmental relationships have changed or remained the same. They are asked to include in their present families and in families of origin whomever they will. Animals are sometimes included, quite often with much significance! It is remarkable how much information comes through in these family drawings, as I hope you will see through this case study of a very pained and despondent adolescent. Before I go into his story, however, I want to give a more cogent and systematic rationale for the psycho-spiritual assessment.

The value structure of many individuals is intimately linked to their religious feelings, images and beliefs. This is so, whether or not these feelings, images and beliefs are positive or negative with regard to religion or God. Understanding an individual's religion or non-religion can illuminate his/her psychological profile and hence facilitate therapy. If there is no specific inquiry about a person's religion or spirituality, that individual may not spontaneously express these matters, thus missing a possible avenue for therapeutic understanding and change.

Just this past year I was called to consult on a case of a woman with depression who had been hospitalized for a month and who had made little or no progress. We had two sessions and I reported to the psychiatrist what we had talked about and my observations, thinking that there was nothing new or particularly unusual in what she had told me. On the contrary, I discovered that she had not mentioned some emotionally significant events to him. She had not told him she had recently experienced a religious conversion, that as a consequence she had stopped acting out sexually, and she was no longer expressing her frequent rage as she had done in the past. In other words, she had locked the psychiatrist out of her "religious life." Suppressing her rage and her rather promiscuous sexual activity were "religious issues" not to be discussed with a psychiatrist.

When the psychiatrist said he knew nothing about this change in the way she dealt with her anger and her sexuality, issues surely pertinent to her present depression, I went back to her and asked, "Why didn't you mention these matters to him?" She said, "Well, he wasn't born again." That answered it for her. I had in no way indicated that I was "born again," but I was someone who had a religious identity as well as a psychoanalytic one, so she felt free to talk about religion. She perceived the psychiatrist to be totally "secular," and one did not talk about sacred matters with him. It was a dramatic instance of a very important matter relating to her depression, but one she thought could not be appropriately resolved in the context of "secular" psychiatry.

Recent studies in object-relations theory have indicated that a person's image of and feelings about God are formed out of complex elements from the whole early parental interaction. Unlike the way Freud saw it, religious development does not for all practical purposes begin and end with the resolution of the Oedipal complex. An understanding of the whole development of a person's God image and the changes which that image has or has not undergone is important and provides valuable insight into a person's developmental issues.

Care must be taken that a spiritual assessment should not be considered a judgment of a person's spirituality; rather, its purpose is to explore whether or not and to what extent a person's spirituality is syntonic or dystonic with other psychological processes. Aspects of a person's spirituality or religion that are ego dystonic can be brought to the person's attention and his/her cooperation can be sought to explore, utilize, develop, and, when necessary, confront their spiritual and religious perceptions and understanding.

Mental health professionals often overlook the fact that there are developmental resources in the various religious and spiritual traditions that properly trained religious professionals are able to bring to bear for the individual's and the family's growth. These resources are variously called pastoral counseling, spiritual guidance, or spiritual direction, etc. They involve an understanding of the criteria of religious and spiritual growth and of religious and spiritual aberrations, and how to encourage the one and how to deal with the other.

One of the unfortunate results of the split between science and religion in general, but more particularly for our purposes, between psychiatry and religion, is that the vast resources of our spiritual traditions have been cut off from the storehouse of both psychiatry and psychology. Spiritual resources, therefore, have been consequently cut off from the patients who consult psychiatrists, psychologists, analysts, and other mental health professionals. Both religion and psychiatry are realizing that neither is omnipotent or omnicompetent and that their professionals need to talk with one another for their own sakes and particularly for the sake of the patient.

In general it has been recognized that a patient's lack of knowledge about his/her therapist's religious belief or disbelief may facilitate the freedom of the psychotherapeutic interchange and mitigate certain transference obstacles. But that lack of knowledge can also make it difficult, if not impossible, for the therapist to facilitate and utilize a person's religious resources to facilitate personal change. An appropriately trained religious professional, aware of the possible misuse of religion to escape issues, can use religious and spiritual resources precisely to facilitate confrontation of important issues and hence remove obstacles to growth. The case I am going to present to you is such a case.

Many mental health professionals recognize their own limited knowledge about religion and perhaps have not worked through their own religious and spiritual issues. Therefore, they are not in a position to inquire about and effectively help resolve another person's religious conflicts because of the counter-transference issues which would arise. Often, then, mental health professionals, wisely, do not inquire into this area of a patient's life. But for many patients that leaves an important psychologically relevant area of a patient's self-understanding inadequately understood. This is a particular problem in a hospital setting since the hospitalized patient does not have easy access to religious professionals.

In addition, mental illness and hospitalization themselves can raise profound issues of personal value and meaning. For many patients hospitalization is the greatest crisis of their entire lives. Not to make religious professionals knowledgeable and sensitive to psychotherapy, available to those patients who desire it, deprives them of a significant resource in coping with the present crisis of their mental illness and hospitalization.

The aim of psycho-spiritual assessment and the possible involvement of clergy in the therapeutic process is not in itself to promote religion. Rather, it is to recognize that, for many persons, religion is an integral part of life and a resource for facilitating personal growth. Religion has nothing to lose and much to gain from psychotherapy's effects on the neurotic elements people take into their religion. Psychotherapy has nothing to lose and much to gain from religion's contributions to personal growth.

Let us turn now to the case I want to describe to you. I first began working, not with the thirteen-year-old black adolescent whom I will call Mike, but with his mother. His mother, a 34-year-old black woman whom I will call Doris, was in the hospital for depression and awaiting the results of an HIV test. Her husband had died from AIDS six months prior to her hospitalization. It was typical of Doris' pattern of denial that she had not been tested for HIV before. She also had an eating disorder and was quite overweight.

In the drawing of her original family, Doris drew herself as a girl with her hand up in the air. She was the "tomboy" in the family. She stated that she wanted contact with her daddy, but did not get it. Her drawing shows this. Their hands do not touch. She felt Daddy fed and clothed them but he was not there for emotional support. I did not meet Doris' sisters, but others who had met them described them as very slim and well dressed. The mother, whom I did meet, was somewhat disheveled.

Doris was clearly a very bright woman with a sharp sense of humor and could draw quite well. Rarely would she directly acknowledge anything positive that had taken place in the therapy, but her appreciation would come out indirectly when she delighted in telling me the advice she generously gave to other patients. The reflections she gave them were invariably the reflections which I had made to her. The focus of my religious work with her was on her anger at God, at her parents, and at her deceased husband.

In speaking about her drawing of her original family she described feeling angry. She portrayed that anger as dark lines on her father's shirt and surrounding her parents. Her father almost looked like a Frankenstein figure. She described her mother, drawn with vacant eyes and a disengaged expression, as unconnected to anything. When her husband was diagnosed with AIDS and she needed a new car, her father agreed to get her a new car only on the condition that her husband never ride in the car, lest he contaminate it. She agreed to that condition even though it would humiliate both her husband and herself. Doris also lived in a house she rented from her father. Even at 34, she was still in angry dependence on her father.

After marriage to the man I will call Sam, she gave birth to a child, the boy I will tell you about. Following "Mike's" birth, his father left the family and the city for six years. When he returned, they had a second child. It is uncertain when the father acquired AIDS. The father's absence during the first child's early developmental years, needless to say, had strongly affected the thirteen-year-old son. The mother described herself as formerly very close to Mike, although the expression on his face in her drawing of him showed confusion about the relationship, as did a question mark she drew above her head. She drew her husband and the young six-year-old child as being very close to each another. Sam had been home and involved in the youngest boy's upbringing. The drawing she made of her husband was very masculine, emphasizing the fly of his trousers. Doris denied that she knew he was gay or bisexual when she married him. The family, however, said they all knew at the time, so at some level Doris must have known as well. Having grown up with a distant, ineffectual father, at least at far as she was concerned, Doris chose a distant and inadequate husband.

Doris then drew a picture of the family after Sam's death. It portrayed her seated in an armchair. Her six-year-old son was making good grades in school and in the drawing was handing her his grades. Her back was turned in anger to the thirteen-year-old son who was doing badly in school. She said there was such a chair in her house that she would plop into after work.

Although Doris clearly had considerable ability, she worked at a domestic job that did not utilize her capacity. When we got to know each other better and she realized I accepted her for who she was, she began to delight in telling me how she would deal with white people at her job. She referred to it as her "Aunt Jemima routine": when a white person was condescending to her, she would move into her "Aunt Jemima routine" and by acting out stereotype would secretly gain the upper hand in the situation. Her anger was often expressed in passive/aggressive ways.

Her rage against black men was enormous. She confided that when she drove her car and saw a black man, she would try to run him over, actually driving onto a curb or onto the grass to do this. The staff confronted her about the behavior and, to my knowledge, she has discontinued it.

In the drawing of her relationship to God, she drew herself weeping and praying, "Bills, sadness, illness, depression! Please help me." In drawing her relationship to Jesus, she drew herself as kneeling at Jesus' feet. She had Jesus saying, "I am with you." Her posture was significant: the figure she drew was crying in a very humble posture, but a posture with a lot of inward rage, expressed by fragmented black lines on her garment. Doris was very fearful about expressing anger at God. Ironically, the anger at God she was "afraid to express" was portrayed in the drawing as her putting herself in God's position above the drawing of Jesus. There was no image of God; she had replaced God. This inflated view of herself was compensation that gave her self-worth and allowed her to function. If her powerful father was the principal available image to make into the image of God, that drawing indicated she wanted to obliterate her father, God, and replace God with herself.

A couple of weeks after she entered the hospital, her thirteen-year-old son visited her. Mike was in the process of a sixth suicide attempt. At home he had placed a cocked gun to his head and was going to kill himself. Someone discovered him and he was hospitalized. After getting to know him and discovering that he prayed, I asked him to draw his relationship with God. He selected yellow paper and drew a sun with eyes and wrote in the sun "God all good." He described the picture as God smiling at him. But if one covered the "God all good" phrase and looked at the eyes he drew, there was no smile. When I asked him to draw his relationship to Jesus, he drew a hand and he told me, "This is Jesus saying, 'Peace.' " The hand, however, looked like a clenched fist rather than an open hand; it was no less a symbol of his projected rage than the scowling "sun" God.

He drew a picture of his early family and creatively entitled it "Fun Times." He described his dad walking on water at Pontchartrain Beach. At that beach, the water is just about six inches deep, so you can walk quite far out into shallow water. Significantly, he described his dad holding not himself, but his younger brother, with whom there is good eye-to-eye contact. To all appearances, he was not even in the picture "Fun Times." I asked him where he was? He explained that in the lower right corner of the picture was the back end of a car: "I'm in the car with my mother." Later I asked what he was doing in the car with his mom. He disclosed that even at thirteen he was often sleeping in the same bed with his mother at home. "Fun Times," then, was wishing for the mirroring his brother got from his dad, but it was also a time of enmeshment with his mother.

In another picture Mike drew "Bad Times." This was after the death of his father. He drew himself on the bed on which his dad had died. It looked like a sarcophagus. As a dream fantasy, he drew a tombstone with "R.I.P. Sam" for his dad, and he drew a coffin with his own name, Mike. Next to his bed, he drew another tombstone with "R.I.P. AIDS" on it. The "R.I.P. AIDS" recalled for him the actual tombstone of his dad with flowers on it. He also drew two snakes in the sky intertwined. This symbol expressed why he wanted to die–so he could be with his father in heaven and get from his father the sense of phallic manhood that he did not get from him during life. He wanted the healing of his basic self through union with his dad. He could be healed there in the heavens. In this sense, the suicide attempt was partially an act of hope. At one point I asked him if he thought he could get from other people what he did not get from his dad. He said, "Yes, I think I could, but I don't want to."

Later I asked Mike his favorite Bible story. He said David and Goliath. I asked him to draw it because the story's young, apparently weak David was eventually victorious. I thought it could provide a creative image for the therapy. Mike clearly identified with David. Goliath was drawn as tall, big, erect and phallic. David was drawn on his knees, small and bent, how Mike felt at the time. Both David and Goliath wore skirts. Mike did have questions about his own sexual identity and had been sexually abused by a friend of his father.

All of this was very helpful diagnostically. But I feel one need not stop there, as Dr. Rizzuto did in her research. I think we can also do further work therapeutically with the religious imagination and let deeper resources of the imagination provide healing possibilities.

I decided to use Ignatius Loyola's and Jung's method of contemplation and active imagination with Mike. I chose the story of the little children coming to Jesus. I asked Mike to imagine himself going up to Jesus after the others had spoken, and to speak to Jesus about what was on his heart and mind. He said he really could not approach Jesus. The image that came to him was that of a one-room house. He could see Jesus through the window with his back to him. There were two guards guarding the house, one in ancient dress and one in modern dress, and he felt he could not enter. He asked me, "Where do I go now?" and I suggested he take his little brother with him and see if he could then go back and have a talk with Jesus. Mike told me he was unable to do that, too. He believed anyone who looked God in the face would die.

"Mike," I said, "there were two guards in that first image and yet you're the only other person except for Jesus. What are the guards doing?"

"They're defending Jesus."

Then I suggested they must be defending Jesus against him. At first he was surprised, then there was that glint of recognition in his eyes. He began to admit how furious he was at God for having taken his father. The extent of his rage was such that in the hospital one day he went on a rampage, an incident which began when a male attendant in the hospital put his arm on Mike's shoulder. Apparently the gesture raised too many issues for him and he responded with rage.

A couple of weeks later when I saw him, he had improved. He had become more sociable had made friends with one of the girls in the hospital. He had begun to do better in school. Mike was above average in his ability and began to show it. Then one day he came to me and said, "I was able to talk to Jesus today." He explained, "I imagined going into that room and there were two chairs. I sat catty-cornered to Jesus. At first Jesus had his hand over his eyes. However I moved to look, Jesus kept moving his arms so that I couldn't see his eyes. It made me very angry that Jesus was doing that. Then Jesus put down his hands and I looked directly into

Jesus' eyes. Once I looked into Jesus' eyes, all my anger disappeared."

I hear many, many levels in this description. First was the issue of the mirroring, going back to the mirroring that he did not get from his dad, the mirroring he was getting from his peers, from his psychiatrist, and from me. The mirroring was providing some of the psychological base which allowed him to work through some of the religious imagery, and this in turn was helping him work through some of the psychological issues. A week later, he came to me and all he said was one thing: "David's won." He meant he had made the decision to live.

Mike required one additional hospitalization a year later to deal with some of the incestuous issues about his mother. The specific issues with his father occasioned the first hospitalization and the issues with his mother occasioned the second.

REFERENCE

Rizzuto, A.M. *The Birth of the Living God.* Chicago: The University of Chicago Press, 1979.

Response to
"Rage at God and Its Transformation: An Adolescent Male and the Death of His Father from AIDS– An Object Relations Perspective"

The idea of a spiritual assessment and the structure of that, whether it is ego-syntonic or dystonic is fascinating. We could spend a couple of hours talking about it. But I choose to challenge all of you.

I agree with the notion of clarity and distinctions Dr. Gregson advocates. Dr. Gregson knows when he is operating as a therapist. He knows when he is in an atmosphere of spiritual growth. He knows when he is combining the two. And he and the patient/client always know which mode they are in. To me that is extremely important. I am not sure all of us are able to make those same clear distinctions.

The patient made me think of a diagnosis that is rather prevalent in this hospital, that of borderline personality disorder. The diagnosis is usually made in females between the ages of 16 and 30. The aspects of the case that made me think of this disorder were these: identity confusion, often with gender confusion; uncontrolled periods of anger and rage; labile moods; unstable relations in which there is idealization and devaluation; and multiple suicide attempts.

Patients like this are very disturbed. They are usually young women who often have serious sexual and physical abuse in their

[Haworth co-indexing entry note]: *"Response* to "Rage at God and Its Transformation: An Adolescent Male and the Death of His Father from AIDS–An Object Relations Perspective." " Clarkin, John F. Co-published simultaneously in the *Journal of Religion in Disability & Rehabilitation* (The Haworth Press, Inc.) Vol. 1, No. 2, 1994, pp. 79-80; and: *Pastoral Care of the Mentally Disabled: Advancing Care of the Whole Person* (ed: Sally K. Severino and The Reverend Richard Liew) The Haworth Press, Inc., 1994, pp. 79-80. Multiple copies of this article/chapter may be purchased from The Haworth Document Delivery Center [1-800-3-HAWORTH; 9:00 a.m. - 5:00 p.m. (EST)].

backgrounds, although not always, and whose suicide attempts are grotesque. One women I know took herself out into the woods and tried to eliminate herself by setting herself on fire. Other women carve their names or others' names in their legs and calves and cut themselves many times. Dr. Otto Kernberg and we who work with him have developed a treatment that is a modified, psychodynamic treatment specifically for this disorder. We are trying to research that treatment and to teach young professionals in mental health how to do it. It is of primary concern that our treatment be geared to the specific disorder. We try to be very clear about our theory of the disorder's genesis, about the prognosis and the natural course of the disorder, and in teaching about it. We have a book that describes the treatment in detail and video tapes showing experts like Dr. Kernberg actually doing the treatment. Students are filmed during therapy sessions and their performance is consistently evaluated to assure that the therapy is done as described. Why am I telling you this? It is a challenge. I think we should meet again a year from now and at that point I would like to see a manual describing spiritual counseling.

John F. Clarkin, PhD

Response to
"Rage at God and Its Transformation: An Adolescent Male and the Death of His Father from AIDS– An Object Relations Perspective"

Dr. Gregson's presentation was clearly a demonstration of talking about the dystonic conflicts and affects within this child, and looking at them through the religious material in order to understand them, acknowledge the affects, and bring forth an understanding of the conflicts. His point is critical. As we are able to create an environment where people feel free to talk about their deepest beliefs, we are often able to see their deepest longings, conflicts and affects and to help them to express those.

In the program I direct at the Blanton-Peale Graduate Institute, the residency program is aimed at training clergy, religious professionals and people who want to integrate counseling and spirituality in psychoanalytically/psychodynamically-oriented psychotherapy.

One course within our program is based on the work of Ana-Maria Rizzuto. In it, each resident presents his/her family genogram and talks about how their faith and values have developed out of family background and experiences. They look at their god-image as distinct from the God beyond God. Often, at the beginning of this course, residents confide in the teacher a real hesitancy to get involved, and may want to decline participation in the class, worried

[Haworth co-indexing entry note]: "*Response* to "Rage at God and Its Transformation: An Adolescent Male and the Death of His Father from AIDS–An Object Relations Perspective."" Wyrtzen, The Reverend James C. Co-published simultaneously in the *Journal of Religion in Disability & Rehabilitation* (The Haworth Press, Inc.) Vol. 1, No. 2, 1994, pp. 81-83; and: *Pastoral Care of the Mentally Disabled: Advancing Care of the Whole Person* (ed: Sally K. Severino and The Reverend Richard Liew) The Haworth Press, Inc., 1994, pp. 81-83. Multiple copies of this article/chapter may be purchased from The Haworth Document Delivery Center [1-800-3-HAWORTH; 9:00 a.m. - 5:00 p.m. (EST)].

81

that they will somehow damage their faith. They fear they will lose their faith as they begin to take a look at this evolution of their systems of beliefs and at the god-image they have held up for themselves. Invariably, I am told, at the end of the course, after they have shared their genograms and talked about how their religious faith has evolved out of their whole learning experience, they come back saying, "My faith is stronger because I've done this. I've understood things about myself and I have let go of some things, and I have changed." One teacher of this course would begin by sharing his own genogram and talking about his own spiritual journey. He once told me "Every time I do it, I am amazed that it is different. I realize that I have grown in some way and that what I am talking about has changed and developed in some particular way." When people finish this course, they are ready to do what Dr. Gregson is talking about, to help people look at their god-image and their religious beliefs in a caring but in-depth way, and to recognize that which is dystonic and distorted and to release the affects contained within that; they are able to do so while affirming the things that are important and valuable for the ongoing growth and the religious life.

I appreciate the story of this boy because I, too, have witnessed these amazing experiences. There is a feeling of awe when a client is able to express pent-up anger at God and release all the feelings of anger with honesty and realness, to come forth and say with Elijah, "Lord, thou has been to me a dry brook." (Remember Elijah under that bloom tree, furious about what he has seen happening around him in life?) There is quite a distinction between talking with God and talking to God–saying directly what we are feeling about the life we are living.

One of the residents in our program was telling me about working with an HIV-positive client. The man had been seriously abused as a child by an alcoholic father and was a recovering alcoholic himself. They had been confronting his fear of dying alone, and the aloneness he experiences in his life. At times she had given him spirituality-focused meditations, finding that they helped him to strengthen his trust in her, as therapist present to him, and his trust in God, as present in his life. As he became able to pray about his anger and jealousy, he has felt less afraid of being alone or dying alone, and has experienced a sense of God's presence with him.

Another association I have had is with one of our other programs, a pastor's program in which students develop and pursue a project in their places of ministry. One student developed a project in which she was co-leading a group of HIV-positive, drug/alcohol addicted, indigent men. She had each of them draw pictures at the time they joined the group and at regular intervals afterwards. The pictures were of their disease, their higher power, their healthy selves, and of their addicted selves. As the group progressed, the men worked on expressing what they were experiencing in drawing the pictures. They could see a progression of change in their self-image and in their image of God as they went forward.

If we, as therapists, can be an unanxious presence with our clients as they share their religious material and their religious concerns or pain, we can encourage the person to come forth and the affects to be understood.

The Reverend James C. Wyrtzen, DMin

Mending the Mind and Minding the Soul: Explorations Towards the Care of the Whole Person

Ann Belford Ulanov, MDiv, PhD

CONVERSATION

The two worlds of psychiatry and religion have not always been on the most cordial terms–there has been much mutual accusation and much mutual suspicion. From the psychiatric, and even the depth psychological perspective, religion has been seen as a delusion, a product of infantile wishes projected onto the cosmos. It has been thought to keep us childish, looking for a divine mommy or daddy, and to leave us unable or unwilling to face the harshness of reality and the reality of the unconscious. In addition, religion has been seen as a short-circuiting of ego-functioning. Instead of growing our way to an attitude or a position, religion has been viewed as a ready-made formula picked from a religious tradition. Religion has been seen as augmenting psychotic processes, as tempting the ego to fall into identification with archetypal energies, as offering an eternal mother's lap with instant gratification for pregenital strivings, or as offering ammunition for a punitive super-ego. Religion has been perceived as the weapon of repression, authoritarianism, even of theological sadism, not to mention a great deal of fuzzy thinking.

[Haworth co-indexing entry note]: "Mending the Mind and Minding the Soul: Explorations Towards the Care of the Whole Person." Ulanov, Ann Belford. Co-published simultaneously in the *Journal of Religion in Disability & Rehabilitation* (The Haworth Press, Inc.) Vol. 1, No. 2, 1994, pp. 85-101; and: *Pastoral Care of the Mentally Disabled: Advancing Care of the Whole Person* (ed: Sally K. Severino, and The Reverend Richard Liew) The Haworth Press, Inc., 1994, pp. 85-101. Multiple copies of this article/chapter may be purchased from The Haworth Document Delivery Center [1-800-3-HAWORTH; 9:00 a.m. - 5:00 p.m. (EST)].

The religious perspective is not much better. Psychiatry and depth psychology have been viewed with fear and disapproval. I have called this the "Christian fear of the psyche" (Ulanov, 1986). Psychiatry and related disciplines are criticized as having a materialistic outlook that reduces the person to chemical functioning or at best ego-adaptation while eclipsing the life of the soul. Further, psychiatry and related disciplines are accused of promoting a pseudo-religion of their own in which we no longer think seriously about wickedness or evil, but rather we think about what we are projecting. We no longer think seriously about achieving a life of faith, but instead about achieving a "mature identity." Worse yet, we don't think about making the world a better place, but instead think about how to "get in touch with our feelings."

Much conflict has existed between psychiatry and religion. Hence, it is a momentous effort that is being made here to inaugurate a vigorous, active, ongoing dialogue between the two disciplines. They are not the same, and they should not be collapsed into one another. A gap persists between them which we need to respect and value, for it preserves the space between the disciplines that makes their engagement and conversation possible. The conversation between the two disciplines of psychiatry and religion (which is the name of the Program at Union Theological Seminary) mirrors the conversation that goes on in each one of us between the psyche and the soul, a conversation that is going on all the time, if you will, in Being itself. We can understand, then, why so much resistance to this conversation is exerted from both sides! The conversation between psychiatry and religion echoes something mysterious that goes on inside each of us and at the center of Being.

Theology has known about this conversation at the heart of Being for a long time. There are doctrines that deal with it. For example, in Christian theology there is the doctrine of the Trinity, hammered out through the vigorous controversies in the third and fourth centuries about the nature of God. Christians made the audacious effort to describe what goes on within God when God isn't doing anything, but is just sort of sitting around being. The Trinity is an effort to describe God's inner object-relations, or what happens between God's id, ego and super-ego, or the congress between God's ego and Self. Despite the numerous arguments, all agreed that the inner life of Being is a vigorous, active, spirited, conversation between different persons, i.e., different aspects of Being. Engagement and exchange go on all the time at the heart of Being. We are attempting in this symposium to listen in on this conversation.

The chaos theory is very much on my mind. The chaos theory states that when a butterfly lifts its wing in Chicago, the atmosphere changes in China. Who knows, maybe we are a butterfly wing. Our talking about these matters of psychiatry and religion may make accessible deep resources of Being for people in this hospital complex and people outside of it, too. We live in a unitary world, where body and spirit cohere, inner and outer life meet, individual and community join. What we do with these two disciplines of psychiatry and religion bolsters our inner conversation between psyche and soul and enables us to perceive it going on around us all the time.

When I speak of psyche, I mean the conscious and unconscious processes that enable us or disable us to be a person in the world, in relation to others and to life. When I speak of soul, I mean the willingness to be such a person in relation to self, other, and God. In old-fashioned terms, soul is a place in us that is like a doorway always open, through which God can barge at any moment. It is an unlockable door. From the psyche's point of view, when we take an interest in religious experience, we want to ask how it functions in ourselves, in our group, in our world. Does it breed illness, or does it promote health?

From the point of view of the soul, we ask a different question of religious experience. We want to know, "Is it true?" From the psyche's point of view, when we feel summoned or called by God we ask, "What was this experience like? How do we accommodate it?" But the soul question is, "Who is calling, and what is to become of Thee and me?" In actual life, of course, psyche and soul are intertwined. Oversimplifications are only of limited use, and then only in symposiums, not in living. But it helps to have these two angles of vision in mind when confronted with tough clinical problems.

For example, a man sought treatment because he was compulsively attracted to teenage girls. With a great deal of labor, it was discovered that he had lost his own adolescence. He said, "I put behind me my dreamy, poetic, idealistic yearnings. I put behind me my soul life." He did this to achieve a solid ego as a barrier against the pull of addiction to drug or drink that had afflicted every member of his family. He succeeded. He got a solid ego, a place in the world, a profession, a marriage, and a standing in his community. But the compulsive attraction to teenage girls overcame him. He was amazed to discover that the girls were the age he was when he had cut off his soul life. In this fearful compulsion that made him feel suicidal, a piece of unlived soul was hiding that now came knocking at his door. It was as if he now could afford to deal with the split-off soul-part because he had built up enough ego strength to do so. And now he must include this soul life or it would destroy him through public scandal and scathing self-judgement. He took up again the conversation with the missing part that was interrupted in his teenage years and it benefitted not only himself, but others in the world as well. His treatment took place some fifteen years ago. You will remember that at that time a great rash of teenage suicides occurred on the east coast. By odd coincidence, this man was asked to speak to an auditorium of teenagers about suicide. His ability to connect with their soul-life was so great that for several years he gave a number of these speeches. His inner conversation helped others in their conversations.

In a more dramatic example, a man suffered spontaneous ejaculations whenever he was confronted by a woman holding a baby or a small child. This occurred in the supermarket, on the bus, in social gatherings, wherever. This man was not at all religious, but in the midst of this vexing body symptom, hid an unadmitted, unacknowledged payment of respect to the power of the feminine, and particularly to its Madonna or Holy Mother aspect. It was as if his unacknowledged religious instinct to venerate a power beyond himself expressed itself through this symptom. If he was not going to pay respect consciously, his body was going to act it out in a literal pouring out of his life fluid.

This religious dimension must be recognized one way or another. It wants to step over into concrete life, into some visible form. This means that in training mental health professionals to help people who are mentally distressed or emotionally disturbed, the training must take account of one's own religious life or non-religious life, one's own God-images, one's own complexes around religion. If we fail to do this, this unexamined religious life will adversely affect our countertransference reactions as easily as do unexamined sexual complexes, images, or drives. In training, we must do the hard reading in spiritual and religious texts that we do in psychological texts so we construct a bigger territory to draw upon in our work. It also means we must make the spiritual dimension a part of the whole treatment. It is not something tacked onto the end of treatment like a pretty scarf to embellish a psychological outfit we have worked hard to put together.

The spiritual dimension is to be taken into account in the initial phases of treatment, where we know it proves a very useful part of the diagnostic procedure. Does this person's religious life promote their craziness, or does it promote their health? That is important, but it is not enough. We need conversation with the spiritual dimension all the way through treatment. Remembering that the two disciplines must not be collapsed into one another, that we need exchange between psyche and soul, we realize it is not enough to alleviate symptoms and recover ego functioning: we also need meaning. Religious experiences, like sexual ones, do not always lie on the surface of the conscious mind. They are often hidden in the unconscious, and we feel great resistance to digging them up. It is an essential part of our training to first find this dimension in ourselves before we can reach to it in our clients. When any of us falls ill or subject to troubles of the heart, mind, or soul, we have lost more than our ego functioning; we suffer more than these distressing, vexing symptoms. We have lost our way; we are living in exile. Conversation between parts of ourselves has been blocked or interrupted.

One suicidal woman said, "I feel like a dried up lake, exhausted." After many months of treatment, she finally confided a dream she dreamt before coming to treatment. I am not allowed to quote the dream because she said it was too precious. In general, I can say that the dream represented a picture of how her soul had been murdered. On the plus side, the dream picture gave her the container, the image, to deal with the agony of annihilation. But, on the minus side, she felt her soul had been made extinct. Although she was not a religious person, this dream was a spiritual event to her. To miss that dimension is to confine ourselves to efforts of recovering ego-functioning which is of priceless value but which will not endure if the spiritual aspect is omitted. If we do not already know this, our patients will tell us by their fierce resistance to recovery when the soul is left out.

I am reminded of Winnicott's words about his psychotic patients. He said, "You may cure your patient and not know what it is that makes him or her go on living. It is of the first importance for us to acknowledge openly, that absence of psychoneurotic illness may be health, but it is not life. Psychotic patients, who are all the time hovering between living and not living, force us to look at this problem, one that really belongs not to psychoneurotics but to all human beings" (Winnicott 1971, p. 100). When any of us seek help from a counselor, psychiatrist, therapist, or analyst, we feel a blow to our souls. We feel we are living in such danger that we have to seek out an office or a hospital which will give us a space safe enough to recover. As many of us know, the person who is in the role of helper must temporarily hold the hope for the person who has lost it. Holding the hope means listening in on the person's inner conversation with a center deep inside and a transcendent center far outside. That listening creates a space for the conversation to be resumed.

This spiritual dimension of clinical work is real and cannot be faked. It is not mumbo-jumbo; it is not pious phrases. To speak of it in religious vocabulary is the exception rather than the rule. Many psychoanalysts approach this spiritual dimension, but they talk about it in their own psychological vocabularies so that we do not always recognize it as spiritual. Such Freudians as Hans Loewald talk about the space between the archaic primary-process thinking of the unconscious that unifies and the secondary-process thinking of consciousness that differentiates us, and how the conversation between them makes us feel alive and real. Winnicott talks about the space of illusion, the transitional space, where we not only find the self we create and create the self we find, but also where culture grows, including religion. Kohut talks about the elusive self that cannot be defined, that inheres in and transcends the structures of the psyche, and without which we do not feel alive. Klein talks about the space between recognizing our aggression and the springing up spontaneously of our instinct to make reparation for destructiveness. Jung talks about the space between the ego as the center of consciousness and the Self as the center of the whole conscious and unconscious psyche. This space that many analysts recognize is where the conversation occurs between psychiatry and religion, between psyche and soul, between us and the transcendent.

RUTHLESSNESS

If we acknowledge the spiritual dimension in the mending of the mind and the minding of the soul, what do we talk about? What do we speak of concretely? First of all, this conversation has no ulterior motive; it makes no converts and takes no hostages. There is no sign-up sheet; no new committees. There are two disciplines here and a space of exchange. In the exchange we are all trying to listen in, to align ourselves to that mysterious center we experience as transcendent. We may experience transcendence as being outside ourselves, our social events, our world, beyond our finite dimension.

We may experience transcendence as something deep inside ourselves, beyond our ego processes, and in those sacred moments of communication when the transcendent enters ego-consciousness. Or it may be all three meanings of transcendence. But in this conversation, we are concrete. We are not talking about talking to each other. We are not talking about trusting each other. Trust, when it is real, does not come by our putting it on the agenda. If the toilet is backing up, it furthers nothing to discuss with the plumber how we want to trust each other while the toilet overflows. Trust comes in this conversation between two disciplines as it does with the plumber. It comes as a gift, a by-product of working together on the concrete problem at hand, clearing the blockage, opening a space for free flow. So what are concrete meeting points in this conversation between psychiatry and religion, between mental health and the life of the soul?

The first is the fact of ruthlessness. We all know the devastation wreaked by mental illness and emotional distress. Minds break up into little pieces and no glue can stick them together again. People turn to stone, inert, dense to any breath of feeling. People are invaded by archetypal energies and feel compelled to act with violence toward self or others. To address such illness we need brute, ruthless strength. I don't mean ruthless in the technical sense of lack of regard to consequences for self and other. I do mean ruthless in the colloquial sense of primordial aggression and the capacity to use it to sustain a long treatment, to yank somebody back from the precipice of suicide, to remain intact before the blast of a negative transference, to risk taking somebody off medication, to persist in concentrated focus on the best self of the other person. We need ruthless strength to pull, push, woo, receive and support that best-self in our analysands which always returns us to our best-self.

I think, for example, of the work of Marion Milner. In her book, *The Hands of the Living God,* she reports her experiences of 22 years of treating "Susan." Susan presented herself at the first session saying that she had lost her soul and that the world was no longer outside her and that all of this had happened since she had received ECT (Milner, 1969, p xix). Milner hung on and very slowly Susan grew a unit-self. But it would not have happened if Milner has not processed her own unit-self right there during all those years. For Milner to do this, she needed to know all about what she described in a later book called *On Not Being Able to Paint.* There she explored "the angry attacking impulses" that are an essential part of a person, "the monstrous creatures" that represent parts of ourselves, the desires "to attack and destroy frustrating authorities," "the wolfish appetites" that cannibalistically devour the other (Milner, 1979, pp. 41, 45, 46, 63). This is ruthlessness.

Closer to home, consider the writings of the Medical Director of this hospital, Otto Kernberg, who reminds us to see others as other, neither merging with them as in the borderline conditions nor treating them as a gas tank to fill up our needs as in the narcissistic disorder. A narcissistic disorder will not be healed by empathy alone. We must use aggressive energy actively to dismantle the pathological grandiose self, and with the borderline condition, we must actively and aggressively limit the patient's acting-out in the world and his acting-in the transference. I see love in this work, but it is love with teeth.

Religion knows all about such ruthlessness and who calls us into it. This is the Christ who comes with a sword as well as peace. This is the Christ who says leave your father and mother, leave your fields and houses to follow me, who calls us to differentiate from our parental images, from our cultural values and find our own way to the center. This means knowing that we are known, and using our aggression to gather all the bits of ourselves so that when the Lord calls we can answer with Samuel, "Here am I." Without reaching this level of aggression, religion degenerates into Mary, meek, mild and powder blue, and Jesus who is pink. In the Hebrew Bible a ruthless Yahweh says, "Come, I am going to make you a people, and I am going to mark out the territory with the law, with the commandment. Take it or put yourself outside this alliance." In Buddhist meditation a Roshi comes to whack between our shoulder blades to make sure we are not just drifting and dreaming, but instead making our way in a precise spiritual direction to the All. This journey directs us to the center. It is not just cozy chats with the Holy.

Ruthlessness also figures at the other end of the health spectrum: we need brute strength to survive integration. Winnicott points out the terrific anxiety that accompanies integration. We define who we are as self, distinct from all those persons and forces now defined as not-self. Unconsciously we expect attack from them (Winnicott, 1988, pp. 117, 119, 121). To be healthy means we are slightly depressed because we are aware of the inevitable mixtures of bad and good in ourselves as well as others. It takes aggression to be responsible for all our feelings, the bad as well as the good, and to hold these opposites together (Klein, 1975, Jung 1959, para. 70-77). Religion knows about this struggle, and knows that integration is not perfection. There is no perfection here below. There is no utopia. That only leads to splitting and violence, where all the good guys are in the corral and all the bad guys are outside to be persecuted, like a borderline condition writ large. Integration means bringing all the bits together, whether in a social community or in a psychic economy. It is a process of struggle and it always lands us in ambiguity, and in surprise.

Remember the parable of the sheep and the goats. Jesus describes how the sheep get saved and the goats damned. The big surprise is that those who thought they were goats turn out to be sheep. They ask, how can this be? Jesus explains that in as much as we visit those in prison, clothe the naked and feed the hungry we have done it for him. In this huge hospital complex and in all the different kinds of work that are represented at this symposium, there are goats who will turn out to be sheep. In this work, you are visiting people imprisoned in their obsessions. You are helping to clothe those naked of defenses. You bring food from the center to those starved for love. But the outcome is never perfect. It is always ambiguous because the transcendent is too big for our finite containers. Religion recognizes with tough-mindedness that ambiguity is the inevitable state of symbols and events where the infinite manifests in the finite. This is not fuzzy thinking or sentimental feeling. When the transcendent takes a small bit of the here and now to show itself, it is always capable of being seen as madness or as stunning revelation. This ambiguity is fact, and it requires ruthless strength to tolerate it.

FATE–DESTINY–PROVIDENCE

Another topic for our conversation is fate, destiny and providence. The suffering of persons who seek psychiatric confinement, or the suffering of those who seek psychoanalysis, psychotherapy or pastoral counseling, is not just discomfort, nor even just dysfunction. Most often it is agony. In places of agony, we lose the thread of our inner conversation. It is interrupted. Sometimes it is made mute. That is why in every city of our country you will find people yelling on the street corner, having imaginary conversations with God or their enemies or you, a perfect stranger walking by. The conversation between ego and deeper Self is so basic to living that when it is interrupted, it will be displaced and transferred into a fantastic dimension. Sometimes it is transferred into the body.

Joyce McDougall writes of psychic deprivation that manifests in severe psychosomatic disorders. Our earliest anxieties and the deepest psychotic layer of our anxieties do not reach words to contain them, nor dream images to express them. They do not even achieve psychoneurotic symptoms to release them. Our missing conversation with this level of our anxiety falls onto organs of the body, and the body must express it in myriad, chronic, obstinate psychosomatic sufferings (McDougall, 1989, p. 53). It is especially poignant when this conversation through body symptoms falls not into our body, but the body of our child.

Many years ago, I treated a woman who after many months of work slowly confided secrets she had held for years. What brought her to treatment was not her secrets, but her youngest child who had been suffering chronic constipation from birth for which no organic cause could be found. The child was four years old when the woman sought treatment. His body carried on the stopped-up conversation of his mother. Gradually, as she let go of her secrets, about prostitution to pay off debts to loan-sharks and gangsters, incurred by her husband's compulsive gambling, and about the paternity of this youngest son, her son's constipation disappeared. He said to his mother, "Don't worry, Mommy. I'm going to be all right. I can let go now." As she began conversation with these mute anxieties, bringing them into words, the little boy's body was released.

People who suffer agony, people who suffer deprivation of soul, who suffer obstinate body symptoms, feel fated. When we feel fated, we feel caught. We need to find places like this hospital, or any resource to recover a sense of destiny as opposed to fate. Christopher Bollas talks about our destiny drive, which he defines as a capacity to generate a future (Bollas, 1991, pp. 47-48). We see from the rioting in Los Angeles in 1992 what bursts into society when people feel they have no future. Wild anger, protest, destruction burst out when we feel fated, when that inner conversation has been foreshortened.

Religion knows about this loss of hope. It knows about our need for a neighbor listening, so that we can find our conversation again. It knows about our need for God as the silent witness to our truest self. Religion knows about the God who is with us in all our hells, in all our cesspools of conflict. Sometimes it is religious experience itself that restarts our conversation. For example, a student took clinical pastoral education (CPE) in a big, crowded city hospital. Mentally ill people were brought in off the street; violence frequently occurred in the emergency room, and there were rows and rows of crack babies lying in their tiny cots looking like little old men and women, shaking, not making a sound. Their parents did not want to see them or to pick them up, but just left them there. One morning, halfway through her course, she got up to go to work and found herself crying and unable to stop. She had the wit to call a friend. Her friend had the wit to hear what was going on and found her a refuge by arranging admission to a private hospital. In a psychodrama session, a profound experience happened to her. The leader suggested, "Now talk to God. Imagine you're talking to God, and tell God what's up, why you're here." She began by describing the crazy people, the violence, the crack babies and how, as a chaplain, she wanted to help and love the poor. Suddenly it poured out of her mouth, "I hate the poor! I hate their indifference, their cruelty! I'm in a rage about it!"

From the psychological perspective, she uncovered the pent-up aggression she had outlawed and made homeless by putting a religious maxim over it that demanded she "love" the poor. Separated from her aggression, she felt helpless and exhausted. Reconnecting with her aggression initiated a theological conversation in her about the necessity of aggression if we are to do any loving at all. The psychodrama leader went further, suggesting, "Okay, now you be God and answer what you yelled." The student was astonished when she heard herself speaking as if she were Christ: "You don't have to sacrifice your life, for I have already made the sacrifice, the last sacrifice. I weep if people don't take this love. But, I have made the last sacrifice." The student felt she found not only her own aggression, but also toughness in God's love. After taking a day or two to digest this, she checked herself out of the hospital, returned to her CPE placement, and finished her work.

Religion reminds us that the sacred is a structure of the psyche. Religion is not an add-on, and not just a helper in making initial diagnoses, but is going on all the time, from beginning to end. Religion takes further the sequence of moving from fate to destiny. The CPE student felt caught in a fate and felt the fatedness of people in the hospital. What she recovered was a sense of her own destiny, and a capacity to listen for its thread in the life of the people whom she confronted in the hospital.

Religion takes us even further in recognizing that we cannot live from the ego-world alone, that even in the most dire straits we must recognize the transcendent element. We discover that even though we seem to be going only back and forth between our problems, that actually, like a sailboat tacking across a waterway, we are creating a path. Discovering this line of destiny opens us to see that the transcendent is touching us, now through a problem, now through a symbol, now through an outer event. Religion tells us that the line from fate to a sense of destiny goes on unfolding into a sense of Providence: that we make a difference, that we matter to what matters. This is not a childish wish, but a theological fact.

Jung describes how we experience the transcendent as an element outside us working in us. In its transcendent function the psyche spontaneously goes back and forth between opposing points of view. We can augment this process by consciously entering it and imagining conversation between our ego perspective–what we want or wish or need–and the perspective of the unconscious that threatens to overwhelm us through a depressive or anxious mood, through a fit of anger or grandiosity, or through a burst of energy or inspiration. As the two sides converse and confront each other, gradually (and with much effort to sustain the dialogue) a third point of view arises spontaneously that includes and surpasses the two opposing ones. It may come as a new image or attitude or insight. Whatever form it takes, it impresses us profoundly. It feels like a solution or a path marked out "in accord with the deepest foundations of the personality, as well as its wholeness; it embraces conscious and unconscious and therefore transcends the ego"(Jung, 1964, par. 856; June 1960, para. 131-193; Jung, 1963, para. 753-756). I would add that through this building up of a third point of view that transcends the ego, we feel the Transcendent touching us, and maybe even guiding us (Ulanov, 1992, Ulanov, 1975, Ulanov, 1982). That which seems far outside us seems to touch, through this process, deep inside us.

When we take seriously the sacred as a structure of the psyche, it introduces a different kind of knowing, one that realizes the limits of ego. It does not replace consciousness. We are driven to use paradoxical language. We move into a knowing that is an unknowing. It is a knowing about deep levels of experiencing that makes our defenses more porous, that softens the lines of separation between subject and object, self and other. It makes our ego more transparent. Some of us call this a feminine mode of knowing, but whatever we call it, this knowing-unknowing paradox introduces us to conversation between ego and archaic mind, between psyche and soul, bringing us to a new level of discourse with our neighbor, including our neighbor God (Ulanov, 1971, pp. 168-193). This is not regression to a pre-oedipal state; it is reaching forward to perception of the unity of Being and Word. It feels free, creative, generative. This is what persons come looking for. If we know it, they will know that we know it, and feel *found*. Fate unfolds into destiny–a line, a path–and we feel breaking in on us a bigger reality, that makes us now see that all along we have not just been unfolding; we have been led. Religion calls this Providence.

SO WHAT?

At this point we might ask, "So What?" And we have all had people in treatment who ask, "So what if I get better? Then what?" Only the determined conversation of psychiatry and religion is tough enough to give the answer: This is the way it is. Like Yahweh told Moses, "I Am Who Is With You" sent you. This God is with us in all our hells and all our happiness. This God, not stuck to one place or to one graven image, is a portable God, traveling above the mysterious mercy seat in the Holy of the Holies within the tabernacle of the Ark.

In the Christian tradition, the answer to, "So what?", comes in person, in the presence of Him Who Is. It does not come in a political program, or in a mental health plan or philosophical concept. The answer comes in person, as presence. And the presence feels big, abundant, like suddenly discovering new budget resources. This abundance feels good. And it is good because it is, as the philosopher Iris Murdoch reminds us when asked what goodness is good for. She replies, "Nothing. Goodness is good for Nothing" (Murdoch, 1969, p. 254).

It usually falls to the lot of those in the conversation between psychiatry and religion to carry this yoke of feeling good for nothing and useless. Despite treatment plans and theories, what are we really doing anyway? Are we doing anything? We often feel foolish, as if we are just sort of hanging out with our patients in the locked ward or in the privacy of our offices. It is not always clear who is the doctor and who is the patient.

What are we doing when we enter this conversation of psyche

and soul, of us and God? We are being; we are present. This is not just nodding to being. We are affirming it. We are not, as a patient once yelled at me "here to get mental health!" What we are doing is getting at the source and giving back to it. This sort of work is unlike any other because it benefits from what does not work. The world of the human psyche and soul is like nothing else because failure is as important as success. We need ruthless energy to see this because this makes fate which strikes us down transform into destiny which leads us to see providence which shelters us. We meditate in this conversation on our failures as opportunities for a success to come. Everybody in this room knows the surprise of finding that it is the wounded place in ourselves that makes the link to the patient, not the developed part of ourselves. Ruthlessly, we meditate on our antipathy, our resistances, our failures, and we do not allow ourselves to be impeded by them. We face the hate and bring it next to the love. A religious realism permits us to do that. We do not lose our compassion when we recognize our hate. We find a basis for it. In this odd work nothing is wasted. We need ruthless energy to go on seeing that nothing is wasted. Everything in our lives is gathered up into the conversation and gives a chance to see God made manifest.

So we who work with the psyche are making an act of faith whether we are religious or not. Our work is not pure science. Its technique is the technique of faith. We work with somebody in ourselves in order to work with somebody in our neighbor. What is given us to live allows us to reclaim all our resources, even our earliest perceptions of the transcendent. This is not regression but a gathering of all our resources. So if we once thought of God as a loving mother who goes on loving us and does not stop just because we got a C − or failed to make the team, we may be able to see now that God does not stop loving us just because we are looters, or crack addicts, or people who put themselves forward as helpers in the mental health profession.

In this profession we have the opportunity to go on with all our resources, both bad and good. And this is where ruthlessness pays off. We are ruthless without doubts, with our incomplete performances because we know they too have a purpose. A woman recently brought this home to me in a fresh way. She brought to her session two or three poems of Rilke's soon after she was released from a hospital in which I had placed her because of a suicidal risk. She was able to gather up this trauma into the thread of her life. She was not religious, but she had a profound conviction that what she had gone through not only was gathered into her own destiny, but contributed to Being itself, and was in an odd way, then, providential. One poem she brought illustrates this (Rilke 1981, p. 175):

> To work with things is not hubris
> when building the association beyond words;
> denser and denser the pattern becomes–
> being carried along is not enough.
> Take your well-disciplined strengths
> and stretch them between two
> opposing poles. Because inside human beings
> is where God learns.

Are we relieved then, of feeling foolish and good for nothing? I'm afraid not. This work pulls us into the center. The ruthless energy it requires can build in us a durability so we can enter into what lasts–like the permanence of a stone, or the redness of red. This ongoing conversation between the disciplines of psychiatry and religion, between psyche and soul within us, that mirrors the conversation going on in Being itself, brings us to the mysterious and inexaustable joy which is always associated with the transcendent. We are not just getting mental health. We are claiming ecstasy, that which builds upon and glows with mental health, that which sometimes has been called spiritual health.

REFERENCES

Bollas, C. *Focus of Destiny, Psychoanalysis and Human Idiom*. London: Free Association Books, 1991.

Jung, C.G. Archetypes of collective unconscious; in *The Collected Works*. New York: Pantheon, 1959.

Jung, C.G. The transcendent function; in *The Collected Works: The Structure of Dynamics of the Psyche*. New York: Pantheon, 1960.

Jung, C.G. Mysterium conjunctionis; in *The Collected Works*. New York: Pantheon, 1963.

Jung, C.G. A psychological view of conscience; in *The Collected Works: Civilization in Transition*. New York: Pantheon, 1964.

Klein, M. On loneliness; in *Envy and Gratitude and Other Works 1946-1963*. New York: Delacorte Press/Seymour Lawrence, 1975.

McDougall, J. *Theaters of the Body, A Psychoanalytic Approach to Psychosomatic Illness*. London: Free Association Press, 1989.

Milner, M. *The Hands of the Living God*. New York: International Universities Press, 1969.

Milner, M. *On Not Being Able To Paint*. New York: International Universities Press, 1979.

Murdoch, I. On "God" and "Good"; in *The Anatomy of Knowledge*. Edited by Grene M. Amherst, University of Massachusetts Press, 1969.

Rilke, M. Just as the winged energy of delight; in *Selected Poems of Rainer Maria Rilke*, trans. Robert Bly. San Francisco: Harper, 1981.

Ulanov, A.B. *The Feminine in Jungian Psychology and in Christian Theology*. Evanston, Illinois: Northwestern University, 1971.

Ulanov, A.B. *Picturing God*. Cambridge, Massachusetts: Cowley Publications, 1986.

Ulanov, A.B. The Perverse and the Transcendent. *Proceedings of the International Congress of Analytical Psychology*, 1992.

Ulanov, A.B. *Religion and the Unconscious*. Louisville: Westminster, 1975.

Ulanov, A.B. *Primary Speech: A Psychology of Prayer*. Louisville: Westminster, 1982.

Winnicott, D.W. *Playing and Reality*. London: Tavistock Publications, 1971.

Winnicott, D.W. *Human Nature*. London: Free Association Books, 1988.

Response to "Mending the Mind and Minding the Soul: Explorations Towards the Care of the Whole Person"

I would like to return to some of Dr. Ulanov's opening comments, in which she said that psychiatry and religion are often very suspicious of each other. I agree. In part, the two fields have been seen as competitors as they sought to explain a similar phenomenon, human behavior. One reason rapprochement between psychiatry and religion is possible today, I suspect, is that both have left the field of battle, at least so far as it affects the seriously mentally ill. I will address my remarks today in an attempt to bring both fields back to what can be a useful battlefield.

The topic today is, "Mending the Mind and Minding the Soul." To some extent, this topic itself is outside the realm of what many psychiatrists would view as the proper domain of psychiatry. Psychiatry has, for better or worse, moved very much towards a biological model where mental illness is regarded as little more than a manifestation of an underlying biological dysfunction. The frequently heard commentary on the move towards biology is that psychiatry, having lost its soul, is now in danger of losing its mind as well. Nowhere is the appeal of the biological greater than in the treatment of the severe mental disorders, manic-depression and schizophrenia. I will present some information about schizophrenia and then return to link it to today's discussion.

[Haworth co-indexing entry note]: "*Response* to "Mending the Mind and Minding the Soul: Explorations Towards the Care of the Whole Person."" McCarthy, Richard. Co-published simultaneously in the *Journal of Religion in Disability & Rehabilitation* (The Haworth Press, Inc.) Vol. 1, No. 2, 1994, pp. 103-106; and: *Pastoral Care of the Mentally Disabled: Advancing Care of the Whole Person* (ed: Sally K. Severino, and The Reverend Richard Liew) The Haworth Press, Inc., 1994, pp. 103-106. Multiple copies of this article/chapter may be purchased from The Haworth Document Delivery Center [1-800-3-HAWORTH; 9:00 a.m. - 5:00 p.m. (EST)].

103

Schizophrenia is a severe mental illness characterized by hallucinations, delusions and disordered thinking. It is associated with profound disturbances in behavior, and for many afflicted individuals, a lifetime of significant deficit and disability. There is abundant evidence that major manifestations of schizophrenia are attributable to the dysfunction of a variety of chemical pathways in the brain. The current operating hypothesis within psychiatry is that alterations of some of these chemical pathways lead to the illness, and that medications which modify these pathways can ameliorate symptoms. It is hard to deny this argument. It is stunning to see the alterations in beliefs and behavior when these severe illnesses are medically treated. These alterations include changes in the thinking process, beliefs, capacity for work and affective state. Moreover, when medications are discontinued, relapse is frequent. The evidence supporting the biological model of schizophrenia is so persuasive that it would be regarded as unethical to withhold biological treatment in almost any study of schizophrenia. Obviously in the past, many of the phenomena described in the severely mentally ill could have been seen as falling within the domain of religion, be it visions or possession. In this battle, psychiatry has apparently won. In fact, some have suggested that modern liberal religions have abandoned the severely mentally ill to secular psychiatry, believing that the care of these individuals is outside the purview of religion (Fink and Tasman, 1992). Is this true?

Psycho-educational treatments have evolved which emphasize the biological roots of schizophrenia. These valuable treatments teach that the illness and its consequent behavior are not so much caused by people but are things which happen to people. This teaching has done much to remove the burden of inappropriate guilt from patients and their families. But these treatments also open the possibility for what Dr. Ulanov has described as "soul murder." To explain to a patient in a psycho-educational model that their illness is a function of a lesion in the brain and that they have limited control over that lesion, certainly can alleviate inappropriate guilt, but it does not empower the individual with the illness. Rather, it can do much to encourage a kind of passivity and helplessness which cannot be restored by our biology. In the attempt to mitigate needless guilt, we can inadvertently reduce the sense of one's self as an active, capable person in the world. Put differently, we can destroy hope and therefore limit the capacity for recovery (Deegan, 1988). I would suggest that biological psychiatry overstates its case and the nature of its victory in the battle in the treatment of the chronic mentally ill. It is true that many of these people respond to medications. But not everyone responds, and, of those who do, few respond in such a way to be said to be fully recovered. Residual disability is commonplace, if not the norm. The work, then, of psychiatry beyond the pharmacological alteration of the brain is in the minimization of disability and the promotion of recovery. This is also the potential locus of cooperation between psychiatry and religion.

Wing and Morris (1981) describe three types of disability within severely mentally ill patients: those that stem from the illness itself; those that stem from the individual's experience of the illness; and, finally, those that result from society's response to these afflicted individuals. Disability stemming from the illness can begin to be addressed by the use of pharmacological agents. A reduction in demands placed on an individual who is biologically incapable of meeting those demands can be addressed by psycho-education. But, as Wing and Morris point out, secondary disabilities may present as much a problem as the illness itself. In these latter disabilities, both psychiatry and religion can and should cooperate. Both of these fields can address in different ways an individual's experience of the illness and of the changes it has wrought. Moreover, both psychiatry and religion are a part of the society whose inept response to these individuals helps to maintain them as disabled. It would be useful to end this inept response. Religion should re-enter the care of the chronic mentally ill knowing full well that such collaboration will be difficult.

In Ovid's *Metamorphoses*, Phaeton extracted from his reluctant father, Apollo, the opportunity to drive the chariot of the sun. The youth, unaware of the difficulty of the task and of his own limitations, raced the chariot upward where his capacities to control his limitations failed. He fell to his death and his family was consumed in grief. Thereafter, his sisters were changed to trees and their continued tears became the jewel, amber. This story applies to both psychiatry and religion. Phaeton's great error was not so much in his aspirations, but in his lack of awareness of his limitations. Likewise, a potentially beneficial collaboration between psychiatry and religion can be damaged should either field give itself over to triumphalism, a sense that one possesses the complete truth untempered by a knowledge of one's limitations. Both fields have been guilty of triumphalism, and both have much to learn from each other.

Richard McCarthy, PhD, MD

REFERENCES

Deegan, P.E. Recovery: The lived experience of rehabilitation. *Psychosocial Rehabilitation Journal* 11: 11-19, 1988.

Fink, P.J., Tasman, A. *Stigma and Mental Illness*. Washington DC: The American Psychiatric Press Inc., 1992.

Wink, J.K., Morris, B. Clinical basis of rehabilitation; in *Handbook of Psychiatric Rehabilitation Practice*. Edited by Wing, J.K. and Morris, B. Cambridge: Oxford University Press, 1981.

Response to
"Mending the Mind and Minding the Soul: Explorations Towards the Care of the Whole Person"

An exploration of the topic, "Mending the Mind, and Minding the Soul" places us in a fascinating position in relationship to the dialogue between psychiatry and religion. I have found a helpful description of this position as a "boundary situation" similar to that of Paul Tillich in his 1936 (later revised in 1966) autobiographical essay, *On the Boundary*. He writes:

> The boundary is the best place for acquiring knowledge . . . since thinking presuppose(s) receptiveness to new possibilities, this position is fruitful for thought but it is difficult and dangerous in life. (Tillich, 1966, p. 13)

The "boundary situation" between psychiatry and religion provides a nearly endless source of intellectual ferment even as it provides innovative and practical approaches to helping others.

Where and how does this "boundary situation" between the disciplines become, in Tillich's words, "dangerous to life?" Those of us who share the stimulation of the dialogue and exercise the benefits of its applications, share responsibility for looking out for inherent problems as well.

[Haworth co-indexing entry note]: *"Response* to "Mending the Mind and Minding the Soul: Explorations Towards the Care of the Whole Person." " Hart, Rev. Curtis W. Co-published simultaneously in the *Journal of Religion in Disability & Rehabilitation* (The Haworth Press, Inc.) Vol. 1, No. 2, 1994, pp. 107-109; and: *Pastoral Care of the Mentally Disabled: Advancing Care of the Whole Person* (ed: Sally K. Severino, and The Reverend Richard Liew) The Haworth Press, Inc., 1994, pp. 107-109. Multiple copies of this article/chapter may be purchased from The Haworth Document Delivery Center [1-800-3-HAWORTH; 9:00 a.m. - 5:00 p.m. (EST)].

I reread recently a short and provocative unpublished address by the theologian, Daniel Day Williams, given at a 1956 meeting formally recognizing the Program in Religion and Psychiatry at Union Seminary. I knew Williams slightly, respected him greatly. I respect him even more now for his understanding of the "dangers in life" of the dialogue between religion and psychiatry.

Williams' piece focused vague thoughts and stated succinctly convictions I have had regarding the issue of language in this dialogue. We know religion and psychiatry share expressions and words that sound the same but may have different implications and meanings. Integration, freedom, guilt, and narcissism or ego-centricity come to mind as examples. Williams asks:

> How are the perspectives behind these two sets of terms related? In what sense do they point to the same realities, and where are the differences between the ultimate perspectives of faith and the psychological structures as science observes and interprets them? What are the ultimates with which we deal when we touch the roots of human action? What is the human spirit? When does psychological healing become a new way of salvation with its own dogma, its ritual, and its charismatic power? Is it a substitute for what the Church means by faith? (Williams, unpublished, 1956)

In our dialogue we rightly recognize idolatry (having false gods) as a shared "danger in life" of our professions. We may see ourselves and others variously as sick, well, estranged, mature, immature, fixated, autonomous. Are our words or concepts our armor, an idolatrous source of power? Are we in danger of becoming modern Gnostics who see ourselves possessing "special knowledge" of eternal wisdom?

Two examples of this sort of abuse came to mind. First, I have seen both parish clergy and chaplains incorrectly use psychological terms and labels to put down (and hence dehumanize) patients and colleagues. I am also greatly disturbed by the uninformed and arrogant use of psychological terms in the process of reviewing candidates for ordination in my own and other denominations. We as persons skilled and interested in the relation of mental health and religion have a special responsibility to monitor these abuses and, where possible, address them. Remaining attentive to this concern entails the "ruthlessness" to which Professor Ulanov alludes.

If there are dangers in living on the boundary, there are privileges of stimulation and promise of greater skills of helping as well. The struggles with boundaries in language, theory, and ethical and philosophical issues of practice are crucial to the dialogue between psychiatry and religion. In that dialogue we must keep in mind what Daniel Day Williams said to us thirty-six years ago:

> Theology and psychiatry converge on the mystery of human selfhood with its misery and grandeur, its hate and love, its despair and joy. A genuinely theological education [and, I would add, all clinical training in the helping professions] will keep its hold on its own distinctive source of insight in its tradition, but it will not isolate itself from the great and profound inquiries into human experience which are now going on. (Williams, unpublished, 1956)

The Reverend Curtis W. Hart, MDiv

REFERENCE

Tillich, P. *On The Boundary: An Autobiographical Sketch.* New York: Charles Scribners, 1966.

Conclusion

The Reverend Richard Liew, PhD

We are still experiencing the effects of the initial hostility with which theologians greeted Freud and the effects, in turn, of his remarks about religion. Nevertheless, within both psychiatric and religious groups there are some who have found harmonization between religious faith and mental health not only possible, but well-nigh inescapable. If progress along these lines is to be made, it will come from those who are willing to lay aside rigid preconceptions in an effort to understand attitudes that may at first sight seem uncongenial to them. Collaboration is a two-way street. It can be blocked by religious thinkers who seize upon popular misrepresentations of psychoanalysis as an excuse for dismissing it without adequate examination. It can also be blocked by psychiatrists and psychoanalysts who hang onto formulae for explaining away all religious belief as illusory, without testing and re-examining their formulae in the light of a wide, sympathetic, first-hand acquaintance with religion at its best.

Both religion and science have something important to say about wholeness and the human condition. Each needs to listen to the other. As Albert Einstein said, "Science and religion now walk hand in hand. Religion without science is blind, and science without religion is lame." Neither religion nor the behavioral sciences has satisfactorily delineated and defined the boundary between them. Yet, as Max Stackhouse suggests, "If one travels far enough in the

[Haworth co-indexing entry note]: "Conclusion." Liew, The Reverend Richard. Co-published simultaneously in the *Journal of Religion in Disability & Rehabilitation* (The Haworth Press, Inc.) Vol. 1, No. 2, 1994, pp. 111-113; and: *Pastoral Care of the Mentally Disabled: Advancing Care of the Whole Person* (ed: Sally K. Severino, and The Reverend Richard Liew) The Haworth Press, Inc., 1994, pp. 111-113. Multiple copies of this article/chapter may be purchased from The Haworth Document Delivery Center [1-800-3-HAWORTH; 9:00 a.m. - 5:00 p.m. (EST)].

111

right direction in one of these areas, he or she inevitably ends up near the other" (Stackhouse, 1975, p. 196). He further suggests that "what happens at the boundaries and the fringes is the center" where fruitful and enriching interchange occurs (Stackhouse 1975, p. 196).

As recent as 1991, the plea for dialogue and collaboration between the behavioral sciences and religion is still heard. This time, it comes from a psychiatrist, epidemiologist, and research analyst from the Department of Psychiatry of Duke University Medical Center (David B. Larson), and an independent science writer who has been widely published in journals and medical textbooks (Susan S. Larson): "Collaboration between mental health professionals and clergy is crucial if those suffering with mental health disorders are to be served more effectively" (Larson and Larson 1991, p. 37).

The symposium, "Mending the Mind and Minding the Soul: Explorations Towards the Care of the Whole Person," is an attempt in a long line of previous efforts in other places to promote dialogue between religion and the behavioral sciences so the best resources of each may be brought to bear upon the process of healing and wholeness of individuals.

This symposium assembled prominent psychiatrists, psychologists, and clinically trained theologians to explore and discuss, through case materials, the interrelationship and intersecting points where each discipline contributes to the objectives of the other. If attendance and favorable responses are valid measures of interest and need, then this symposium definitely confirmed that the need exists for religion and science to be in conversation, and that there is interest.

The publication of this symposium is a consequence of the numerous requests for it to be in print. We owe special thanks to Danika Kapuschansky who took on the tedious task of transcribing the tapes and who patiently retyped the text several times. Special thanks also go to Juliet Goldsmith (Director of Public Information), Diane Clark (Director of Volunteer Services), The Hospital Chaplaincy, Inc., and to the Symposium Planning Committee whose contributions were significant for the success of the symposium. Last, but by no means least, thanks go to the four moderators of the symposium (Rev. Bane, Dr. Bercovici, Dr. Kornfeld and Dr. Silberman), whose eloquent introductions of participants are not included in the manuscript, but whose efforts contributed strongly to the success of the process.

REFERENCES

Larson, D.B., Larson, S.S. Religious commitment and health: valuing the relationship. *Second Opinion* 17: 27-40, 1991.

Stackhouse, M.L. On the boundary of psychology and theology. *Andover Newton Quarterly* 15: 196-207, 1975.

List of Contributors

THE REVEREND J. DONALD BANE, MDiv, MS, is Director of Pastoral Care at the Westchester County Medical Center, Valhalla, New York. He is also a staff therapist, Samaritan Counseling Center on the Shore, Rye, New York and a Diplomate of the American Association of Pastoral Counselors.

THE REVEREND HILLARY R. BERCOVICI, MDiv, PhD, is Rector of St. Mary's Episcopal Church, Scarborough, NY.

HAROLD BRONHEIM, MD, is Assistant Clinical Professor of Psychiatry and Medicine, Mount Sinai School of Medicine, New York City.

JOHN F. CLARKIN, PhD, is Professor of Clinical Psychiatry, Cornell Medical College, and Director of Psychology, The New York Hospital-Cornell Medical Center, Westchester Division.

THE REVEREND TOBY GOULD, MDiv, is Pastor of Memorial United Methodist Church, White Plains, NY.

VERNON J. GREGSON, JR., PhD, is Associate Professor of Religious Studies at Loyola University, New Orleans, and a Senior Psychoanalytic Candidate, Tulane Medical School Psychoanalytic Program.

THE REVEREND CURTIS W. HART, MDiv, is Director of Pastoral Care at The New York Hospital-Cornell Medical, New York City, and President of the Assembly of Episcopal Hospitals and Chaplains. He is a Fellow of the College of Chaplains.

THE REVEREND MARGARET Z. KORNFELD, DMin, is Chairperson (Eastern Region) of the American Association of Pastoral Counselors. She is a member of the faculty of Blanton-Peale Graduate Institute and Union Theological Seminary in New York City and a Diplomate of the American Association of Pastoral Counselors.

THE REVEREND RICHARD LIEW, PhD, is Director of Pastoral Care and Education at The New York Hospital-Cornell Medical Center, Westchester Division.

RICHARD H. McCARTHY, PhD, MD, CM, is Assistant Professor of Psychiatry and Clinical Affiliate of the New York Hospital-Cornell Medical Center, Westchester Division.

H. JONATHAN POLAN, MD, is Associate Professor of Clinical Psychiatry and the Director of Medical Student Education for the Department of Psychiatry, The New York Hospital-Cornell Medical Center, Payne Whitney Clinic, New York City.

SALLY K. SEVERINO, MD, is Associate Professor of Clinical Psychiatry, Cornell University Medical College, and is Associate Medical Director for Program Development and Director of the Evaluation and Admissions Service at The New York Hospital-Cornell Medical Center, Westchester Division.

RABBI JEFFREY M. SILBERMAN, DMin, is Co-Director of Pastoral Care and Education, Lenox Hill Hospital, New York City and President of the National Association of Jewish Chaplains. He is also Director (Eastern Region) of the Association for Clinical Pastoral Education.

THE REVEREND WALTER SMITH, SJ, MDiv, PhD, is Executive Vice President of The Hospital Chaplaincy, Inc., New York City. He is the former Dean and Clinical Professor of Psychology and Pastoral Care, Weston School of Theology, Cambridge, Massachusetts.

ANN BELFORD ULANOV, MDiv, PhD, LHD, is Professor of Psychiatry and Religion at the Union Theological Seminary, Columbia University, New York City. She is a Diplomate of the American Association of Pastoral Counselors.

THE REVEREND JAMES C. WYRTZEN, DMin, is Director of Training at the Blanton-Peale Graduate Institute of the Institutes of Religion and Health, New York City and President of the American Association of Pastoral Counselors.

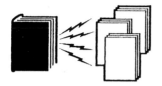

Haworth
DOCUMENT DELIVERY
SERVICE
and Local Photocopying Royalty Payment Form

This new service provides (a) a single-article order form for any article from a Haworth journal and (b) a convenient royalty payment form for local photocopying (not applicable to photocopies intended for resale).

- *Time Saving:* No running around from library to library to find a specific article.
- *Cost Effective:* All costs are kept down to a minimum.
- *Fast Delivery:* Choose from several options, including same-day FAX.
- *No Copyright Hassles:* You will be supplied by the original publisher.
- *Easy Payment:* Choose from several easy payment methods.

Open Accounts Welcome for . . .
- Library Interlibrary Loan Departments
- Library Network/Consortia Wishing to Provide Single-Article Services
- Indexing/Abstracting Services with Single Article Provision Services
- Document Provision Brokers and Freelance Information Service Providers

---

MAIL or *FAX* THIS ENTIRE ORDER FORM TO:

Attn: **Marianne Arnold**
Haworth Document Delivery Service
The Haworth Press, Inc.
10 Alice Street
Binghamton, NY 13904-1580

or FAX: (607) 722-1424
or CALL: 1-800-3-HAWORTH
(1-800-342-9678; 9am-5pm EST)

PLEASE SEND ME PHOTOCOPIES OF THE FOLLOWING SINGLE ARTICLES:
1) Journal Title: _____

    Vol/Issue/Year: _____ Starting & Ending Pages: _____

    Article Title: _____

2) Journal Title: _____

    Vol/Issue/Year: _____ Starting & Ending Pages: _____

    Article Title: _____

3) Journal Title: _____

    Vol/Issue/Year: _____ Starting & Ending Pages: _____

    Article Title: _____

4) Journal Title: _____

    Vol/Issue/Year: _____ Starting & Ending Pages: _____

    Article Title: _____

(See other side for Costs and Payment Information)

COSTS: Please figure your cost to order quality copies of an article.

1. Set-up charge per article: $8.00

   ($8.00 × number of separate articles) _____

2. Photocopying charge for each article:

   1-10 pages: $1.00 _____

   11-19 pages: $3.00 _____

   20-29 pages: $5.00 _____

   30+ pages: $2.00/10 pages _____

3. Flexicover (optional): $2.00/article _____

4. Postage & Handling: US: $1.00 for the first article/

   $.50 each additional article _____

   Federal Express: $25.00 _____

   Outside US: $2.00 for first article/

   $.50 each additional article _____

5. Same-day FAX service: $.35 per page _____

6. Local Photocopying Royalty Payment: should you wish to copy the article yourself. Not intended for photocopies made for resale. $1.50 per article per copy (i.e. 10 articles x $1.50 each = $15.00) _____

GRAND TOTAL: _____

METHOD OF PAYMENT: (please check one)

❑ Check enclosed   ❑ Please ship and bill. PO # _____

(sorry we can ship and bill to bookstores only! All others must pre-pay)

❑ Charge to my credit card: ❑ Visa; ❑ MasterCard; ❑ American Express;

Account Number: _____ Expiration date: _____

Signature: **X**_____ Name: _____

Institution: _____ Address: _____

City: _____ State: _____ Zip: _____

Phone Number: _____ FAX Number: _____

MAIL or *FAX* THIS ENTIRE ORDER FORM TO:

Attn: **Marianne Arnold**
Haworth Document Delivery Service
The Haworth Press, Inc.
10 Alice Street
Binghamton, NY 13904-1580

or **FAX:** (607) 722-1424
or **CALL:** 1-800-3-HAWORTH
(1-800-342-9678; 9am-5pm EST)